Tai Chi Ch'uan & Qigong

Techniques & Training

Wolfgang Metzger & Peifang Zhou
with Manfred Grosser, Ph.D.

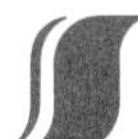

STERLING PUBLISHING CO., INC.
NEW YORK

Credits

All photos by Wolfgang Metzger and Manfred Grosser
Calligraphy by Zhang Youliang
Cover photos by Wolfgang Metzger
Computer graphics by Kartographie Huber

Demonstrators

Peifang Zhou, Lin Boyan, Beijing University of Physical Education; Lü Guangchen, Shan Xiwen, Tai Chi Institute of Physical Education; and Adrian Grosser

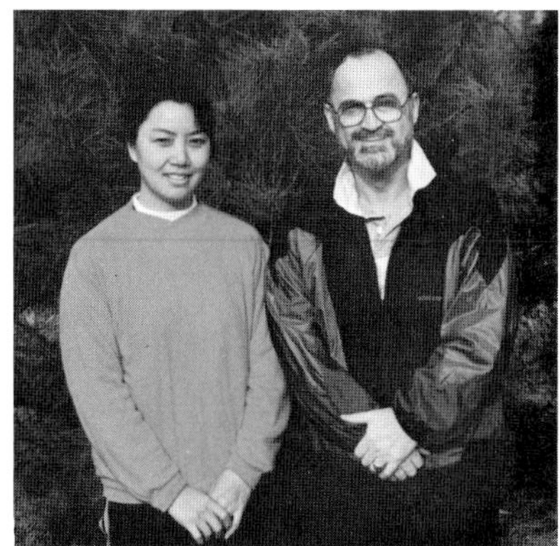

Peifang Zhou and Wolfgang Metzger

In-House Editor Jeanette Green
Translated from the German by Elisabeth Reinersman
Translation Copyedited by Laurel Ornitz

Library of Congress Cataloging-in-Publication Data Available

10 9 8 7 6 5 4 3 2 1

Published 1996 by Sterling Publishing Company, Inc.
387 Park Avenue South, New York, N.Y. 10016
Originally published by BLV Verlagsgesellschaft mbH, Munich,
under the title *Taijiquan Qigong: Der sanfte Weg zu innerem Gleichgewicht und Wohlbefinden*

Distributed in Canada by Sterling Publishing
% Canadian Manda Group, One Atlantic Avenue, Suite 105
Toronto, Ontario, Canada M6K 3E7
Distributed in Great Britain and Europe by Cassell PLC
Wellington House, 125 Strand, London WC2R 0BB, England
Distributed in Australia by Capricorn Link (Australia) Pty Ltd.
P.O. Box 6651, Baulkham Hills, Business Centre, NSW 2153, Australia
Manufactured in the United States of America

Sterling ISBN 0-8069-5957-6

Contents

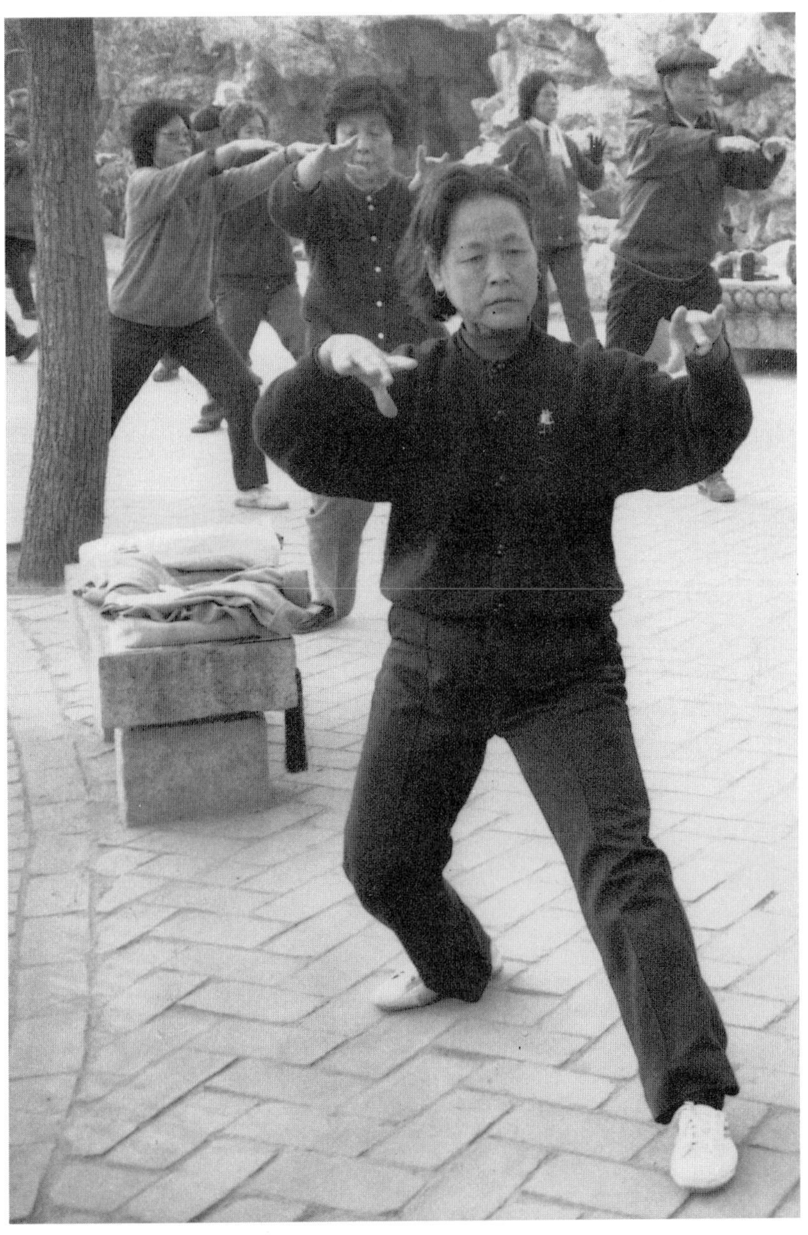

Foreword

This book presents—in words and in pictures—the gentle movements and breathing techniques that make up Tai Chi Ch'uan and Qigong (often transliterated as "Chi Kung"). It is our hope that interested readers will do these exercises every day if their goal is relaxation and a greater sense of well-being. They are an excellent means of stress reduction and the perfect antidote to the hectic pace of modern times, bringing about a more peaceful and, therefore, qualitatively better way of life.

In Chapter 1, we look at the history of Tai Chi Ch'uan and Qigong, showing the influence that traditional Chinese philosophy and thought has had on the practice of body movements and breathing. Chapter 2 will be of particular interest to readers who are looking for a way to consciously slow down the frantic pace of their life, and find more peace and balance. This chapter also discusses the medical benefits derived from practicing Tai Chi Ch'uan and Qigong. Chapter 3 looks at Tai Chi Ch'uan's system of movements, comparing them to those carried out in other sports.

The practical portion of the book, Chapters 4 and 5, introduces a combination of Tai Chi Ch'uan and Qigong exercises, with the Qigong exercises used as a warm-up breathing technique. Of course, the Qigong exercises—precisely because of their excellent therapeutic value—can also be done separately. The Beijing Short Form as well as the Qigong exercises we have chosen are easy to follow and, because of their length and degree of difficulty, won't be too strenuous for the beginner. The simplicity of the Qigong exercises—that lead into Tai Chi Ch'uan—allows you to slowly and carefully become familiar with these unaccustomed movements.

We are, of course, aware that a book can never replace a competent teacher. It should not be too difficult to find a teacher close to where you live; many adult recreational facilities, community centers, and even colleges or universities offer classes.

At this point, I would like to express my appreciation to all who have contributed to this book: first—and most of all—to my coauthor and Tai Chi Ch'uan teacher, Peifang Zhou, and her husband, Lin Boyan, who took on the task of choosing and presenting the Qigong exercises; also to Professor Tian Maijiu, vice chancellor of the Beijing University of Physical Education; Professor Zhang Wenguang, assistant dean of the Chinese Wushu Association; the master calligrapher Professor Zhang Yuoliang from Hangzou; Professor Manfred Grosser, Technical University, Munich; both Liu and Chen Jiaqi, directors of the University of Physical Education in Tianji; and my friends Li Zhenbiao and Mei Hangqiang; as well as my colleague, Hans-Christoph Raab, for all his good advice.

—Wolfgang Metzger

Wolfgang Metzger, born in 1939, studied physical education and English, and was a school principal and a lecturer on physical education. Since 1986, Mr. Metzger has, on a yearly basis, continued his study and training of Tai Chi Ch'uan under Peifang Zhou and other instructors at the College of Physical Education in Beijing. Since 1989, he has taught Tai Chi Ch'uan at the University of Würzburg in Germany.

Peifang Zhou, born in 1954, studied Chinese martial arts (Wushu) from 1974 to 1977 at the former College of Physical Education in Beijing. In 1977 she was the runner-up in Yang Tai Chi Ch'uan as well as the winner of several national titles in other Tai Chi Ch'uan competitions. From 1977 to 1992, Ms. Zhou was lecturer and trainer for Wushu at the College of Physical Education in Beijing. It was during this time that, on the request of the Chinese Government, she also taught Wushu in Japan. Since 1992, she has lived with her husband, Lin Boyan, in Shizuoka, Japan, where both are involved in continuing education. Her husband is pictured demonstrating the Qigong exercises in this book.

In this book, Ms. Zhou's family name is given last for cataloging purposes. Other Chinese names conform to Chinese convention.

Introduction

Everyday Tai Chi Ch'uan & Qigong in China

A tourist in China who is up and about in the early morning hours—particularly on weekends and during the warm months of the year—visiting parks or looking for open spaces in large cities like Beijing or Shanghai will encounter something rather unusual: people converging from different points, some carrying swordlike instruments, gathering in small or large groups and beginning to stretch and flex. After a period of warm-up, they start a series of exercises without the usual huffing and puffing that often accompanies many other exercises. The movements are free of tension and naturally intentional.

Almost every group takes its clues from a leader, often wearing white gloves, who determines the tempo and the sequence of movements and who will, if necessary, correct the participants. Breaks between exercises are filled with pleasant conversations and relaxed humor.

What is it that makes these people do what they do with such dedication and concentration?

Tai Chi Ch'uan at daybreak in Tianjin Park. "Truly renew yourself daily." (Confucius)

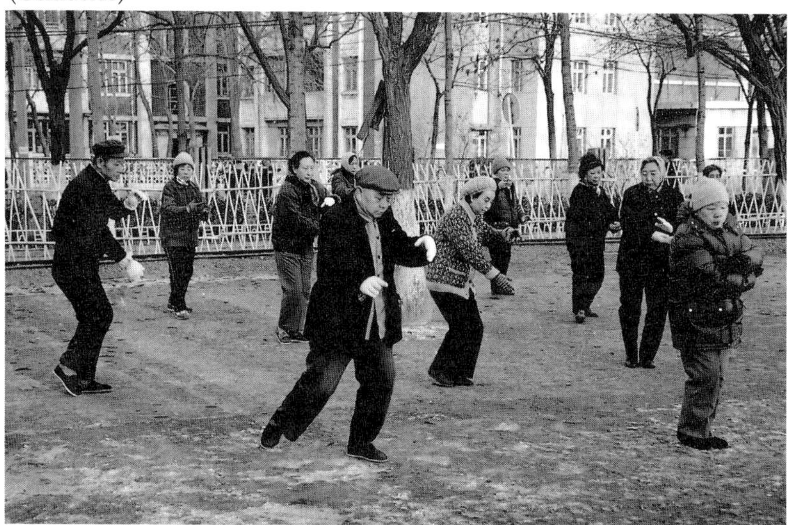

A Poetic Answer

The British writer Aldous Huxley (1894–1963), in his utopian novel, *Island*, creates a picture with words. Qigong, when the novel was published in 1962, was not yet well known outside of China. However, from Huxley's wife, Laura, to whom the novel is dedicated, we know that he was aware of the "dance" of Tai Chi Ch'uan, which he described·

"No leaps, no high kicks, no running. The feet always firmly on the ground. Just bendings and sideways motions of the knees and hips. All expression confined to the arms, wrists and hands, to the neck and head, the face and, above all, the eyes. Movement from the shoulders upwards and outwards—movement intrinsically beautiful and at the same time charged with symbolic meaning. Thought taking shape in ritual and stylized gesture. The whole body transformed into a hieroglyph, a succession of hieroglyphs, of attitudes modulating from significance to significance like a poem or a piece of music. Movements of the muscles representing movements of the passage of Suchness into the many, of the many into the immanent and ever-present One. 'It's meditation in action.' "

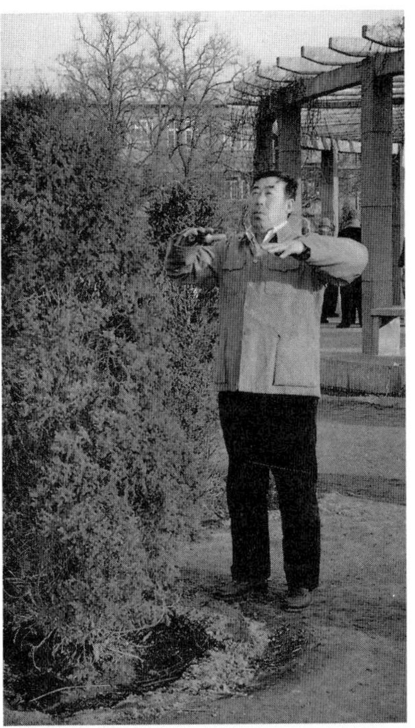

Qigong, drawing strength from nature

Tai Chi Ch'uan & Qigong Today

On one hand, Tai Chi Ch'uan in China today is considered part of the traditional self-defense sport Wushu and is practised competitively. On the other hand—together with the increasing popularity of Qigong—for millions of people in China it has become a very important component for health.

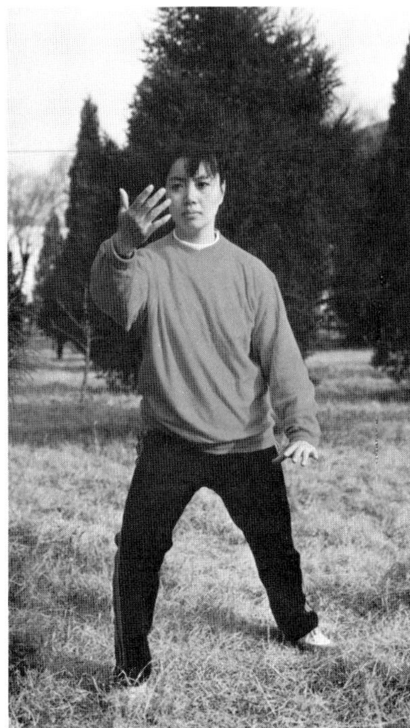

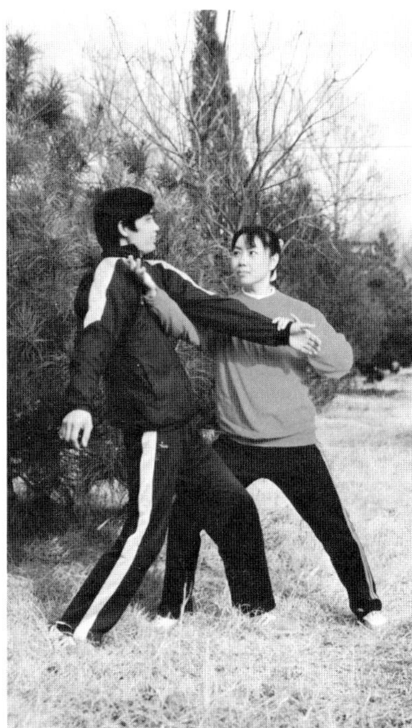

(Left) Form 2 Parting the Horse's Mane and (right) its implementation in self-defense

Tai Chi Ch'uan and Qigong—in the noncompetitive form—is seen as a means of preventing illnesses, stabilizing health, and combating chronic disorders. For a long time both disciplines have been integrated into therapeutic models in hospitals and sanatoriums. To a great extent the social aspect of this activity—getting together with like-minded people in a park or an open space to exercise, to talk, to banter, and to laugh—undoubtedly adds to its therapeutic value.

Tai Chi Ch'uan as a means of self-defense only has importance from a theoretical point of view, but, for a deeper understanding of the individual forms, it should never be ignored. This is because, even in the smallest details of the forms, the basic criteria of the self-defense sport must be fulfilled. The photos above show the connection between the two.

1
Tai Chi Ch'uan & Qigong in Chinese Tradition

History of Tai Chi Ch'uan

Tai Chi Ch'uan as a Discipline of Wushu

In China, Wushu is taught in most universities and colleges that offer physical education, as well as in middle and primary schools. For instance, Tai Chi Ch'uan is a required subject, and involves taking final examinations, for all students at the University of Physical Education in Beijing, Shanghai, and Tianjin.

Wushu consists of a consciously combined sequence of offensive and defensive movements that can be carried out with or without a weapon for self-defense. The weapon could be a spear, stick, broadsword, nine-link chain, or stick consisting of three individual parts joined with hinges.

Tai Chi Ch'uan can also be carried out with or without the use of equipment. When done with a sword or a dagger, it is called either Tai Chi Dao or Tai Chi Chan, respectively.

The most striking difference between Tai Chi Ch'uan and all other Wushu disciplines—for the observer—is the very slow performance of the movements of the former.

Wushu competitions are judged according to a very strict point system similar to that used in gymnastics and figure-skating competitions. The participants "fight" against an imaginary opponent or a sparring partner. Offensive and defensive actions are carried out in a preestablished order, so that direct body contact and, therefore, injuries almost never occur, provided that all rules are adhered to.

At what point Wushu actually became a Chinese self-defense sport is difficult to determine with any degree of certainty. While Tai Chi Ch'uan is at least 300 years old, we know for sure that Wushu is much older. We know, for instance, that as far back as the 7th century—and in many different dynasties—the physical fitness of men who were to be drafted into military service was judged according to their performance in Wushu competitions. We also know that Wushu competitions were supported and carried out in and for the public during the Sung dynasty (960–1279) and the Ming dynasty (1368–1644). During the Qing dynasty (1644–1916), Wushu was promoted as a means of preserving and improving the physical health of the population at large.

In this century, due to both world wars and the political and social turmoil and changes in China following them, the popularity of Wushu beyond Chinese borders did not begin to improve until the 1970s and then again during the middle of the 1980s.

The Establishment of Tai Chi Ch'uan Schools

Tai Chi Ch'uan, independent of Wushu, has its own history: It is the practice of this type of exercise in schools that has preserved and carried on the tradition to the present.

The Chen School

We are, to this day, not quite sure who the true founder of Tai Chi Ch'uan is. In China, people believe that this honor belongs to Chen Wangting, who lived in the 17th century. He was a member of the ninth generation of the Chen family who lived in Honan province.

Chen Wangting drew very heavily from the work of the famous general Qi Jugiang (1528–1587) called the *32 Forms of Fistfighting,* which was the primary instructional handbook at the time for military training. Chen incorporated 29 of the forms into the movements of Tai Chi Ch'uan. For more than 200 years, Chen Wangting's style of Tai Chi Ch'uan was passed down orally from one generation to the next. One of his descendants, Chen Xi (1849–1929), a member of the sixteenth generation of the family, is said to have put together a book over a time span of 12 years called *Tai Chi Ch'uan Illustrated* that is based solely on the Chen style and was published in 1933.

The most famous practitioner of the Chen style in China today is Chen Xiaowang, a member of the nineteenth generation of the Chen family; he has been a national champion in this style several times.

The most distinct characteristics of the Chen style are its smooth, flowing forms that can suddenly change into explosive, jarring movements involving the whole body. Even jumps are part of the overall sequence. Today, a well-known and highly regarded style of Tai Chi Ch'uan is one based on the tradition of the Chen school.

The Yang School

The most popular style of Tai Chi Ch'uan is that of the Yang school. Its founder is Yang Luchan (1795–1872). Born in Yongnian county in Hopeh province, he was from a poor family and came to the Chen family as an apprentice when he was 10. It

The Main Tai Chi Ch'uan Schools & Their Founders

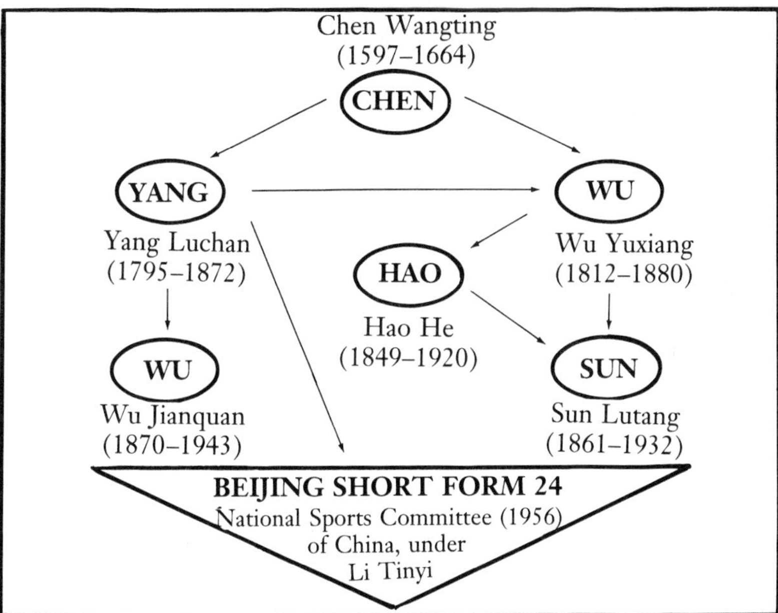

did not take long for his considerable talent in the art of self-defense to be detected. Under Chen Changxing (1771–1872), a master and a member of the fourteenth Chen generation, he became one of the most exceptional Wushu practitioners of his time. At the age of 40, Yang Luchan went back to his hometown, where he earned his living as a Tai Chi Ch'uan teacher. Eventually, he moved to Beijing, where he also taught Tai Chi Ch'uan.

Yang Luchan himself, as well as his son Yang Jianhou (1839–1917), but most of all his grandson Yang Chengfu (1883–1936), were constantly improving and modifying this style. The traditional Yang style, in its basic form, as practised in China today and elsewhere, is based largely on the Yang Chengfu style.

When compared to the Chen style, the Yang style is characterized by especially balanced, flowing movements and the harmonious and seamless way that the transition from one movement to the next is carried out. The movements of this style are also less complicated, which, however, does not mean that they are in any way less effective. The most popular sequences of Yang Tai Chi Ch'uan today are the following:

1 The traditional Yang Form, according to Yang Chengfu (85)
2 The Beijing Short Form (24)
3 The Yang Competition Form (40)

The Wushu School of Wu Yuxiang and the Hao School

When Yang Luchan returned home at the age of 40, he lived on the property of the Wu family. As chance would have it, Wu Yuxiang (1812–1880) met Yang Luchan and asked him to teach him Tai Chi Ch'uan. In order to acquire every minute detail of this form, Wu Yuxiang travelled to Wenxian in 1852 to Yang's teacher, Chen Changxing. Chen, however, due to his advanced age, was not able to teach Wu himself and sent him to one of his nephews, Chen Qingping (1795–1868). He, in turn, taught Wu a revised version of the original Chen style.

Wu Yuxiang, on the basis of what he had learned from Yang Luchan and from Chen Qingping, developed his own style that is characterized by its rapid succession of movements. This style was carried on by his nephew Li Jinglun (1832–1892) and his student Hao He (1849–1920). Hao He later expanded the number of forms within the sequence and added several other changes, which resulted in a new school that carries his name.

The Sun School

During a visit in Beijing, Hao He met Sun Lutang (1861–1932). Sun was from Hopeh province and had developed a reputation in Beijing as a master of the art of fistfighting, called Baguazhang and Xingyiquan. Having become seriously ill during his stay in Beijing, Hao was cared for by Sun Lutang, who also introduced him to the best physicians he could find. In appreciation, when he recovered Hao taught Sun his style of Tai Chi Ch'uan.

Sun integrated what he had learned from Hao into his substantial knowledge of fistfighting and eventually developed the 85 Forms with their own sequences.

The Sun style is characterized by swift hand movements and by the gentle and flowing movements of the legs.

The Wu School

Wu Jianquan (1870–1943) was from a family that originally came from Manchuria. He received his training and gained his extraordinary knowledge of Tai Chi Ch'uan from his father, who had studied under Yang Luchan and his second son, Yang Banhou (1837–1892).

In the beginning, and for many years thereafter, Wu taught the Yang style. Over time, however, he developed a style of his own. In 1928, having been given the title of professor, he taught at the Wushu Society in Shanghai. In 1953 the Jianquan Tai Chi Ch'uan Society was founded, which played a prominent role in the promotion and expansion of the Wu style.

The Wu style is less gentle in its movements; the movements are tighter and the round circular movements are less expansive.

If the different styles were rated, you could say that, after the Yang and the Chen styles, the Wu style—particularly in China—would undoubtedly come in in third place.

History of Qigong

The Chinese have practised various kinds of physical exercise for more than 2,500 years, and Qigong (Chi Kung) holds a special place among them. Integrated into their concepts of philosophy, religion, and medicine of different time periods, including the present, Qigong has almost always been part of supportive therapy and prevention as well as recuperative/rehabilitative care in the Chinese health care system.

Before giving an overview of the history of Qigong, we would like to explain a few repeatedly used concepts. The meaning of *Chi* and *Qigong* is explained in more detail later. However, an often used synonym for *Qigong* is *Daoyin*, which, according to U. Engelhardt, who has written extensively on Tai Chi Ch'uan and Qigong, means a directing and stretching exercise whose aim is to guide the Chi through the body (dao) and to stretch the body (yin), so that the body becomes subtle and allows the Chi to move through it. The abbreviation *TCM* will stand for "traditional Chinese medicine," and it consists of three primary therapies: acupuncture, moxibustion,* and pharmacology.

Its Origins

Before 206 B.C.

• The beginning of the conceptual and philosophical basis of Qigong and TCM: Yin-Yang theory, Five Elements, Chi concept.

• The first written document of Chi exercises, inscriptions in bronze.

• The compilation of the oldest medical writings in the world, the *Huangdi Neijing*, also called *Classical Writings About Internal Medicine by the Yellow Emperor*; included are references to the treatment of illnesses with the Daoyin method.

• The discovery of a nephrite object from the 4th century B.C., with inscriptions of specific Chi techniques.

* Burning certain substances, like mugwort, for instance, above a particular point of the body for stimulation, with the goal of attracting active yang energy.

A Journey through the Centuries

206 B.C.–220 A.D.

• The discovery in 1973 of a silk painting at the Mawangdui tomb No. 3 near Changsha (dating from about 169 B.C.) depicting Daoyin exercises.

• The physician Hua Tuo (about 141–203 A.D.) developed exercises that incorporate animal movements, called the Play of Five Animals (tiger, elk, bear, monkey, bird).

265–419 A.D., Jin Dynasty

• The physician Ge Hong (281–341 A.D.) recommended Chi exercises as a prevention against illnesses and a means of harmonizing the body's energies in his *Prescription in Case of Emergencies.*

581–618 A.D., Sui Dynasty

• The physician Chao Yuanfang (550–630 A.D.), in his *Treatise Dealing with the Origin and the Course of Illnesses*, compiled an assortment of 213 Daoyin exercises for therapeutic use.

618–907 A.D., Tang Dynasty

• A treatise by the twelfth patriarch of the Daoist Shangqing School, Sima Chengzhen (647–735 A.D.), with the title *The Essential Meaning of Receiving Chi*, explained the historic, philosophical basis of the classic Chi exercises and their connection to TCM.

960–1279 A.D., Sung Dynasty

• It is assumed that the term *Qigong* appeared for the first time during this period.

1368–1644 A.D., Ming Dynasty

• A Qigong boom took place during the middle of the 16th century, being used in almost all branches of Chinese medicine. Some of the prominent practitioners were Yang Jizhou (1522–1620), Chen Jury (1558–1639), and Cao Yuanbai (about 1550).

1644–1840 A.D., Qing Dynasty Until the Opium War

• The Qigong boom continued.

• Qigong became the overall term for Chi exercises, establishing itself throughout China at the beginning of the Qing Dynasty.

1840–1911, A.D., Qing Dynasty and Up to the Revolution

• With the decline of traditional Chinese medicine beginning in 1822 following the closing of the Department of Acupuncture and Moxibustion at the Imperial Medical University in Beijing, physicians were restrained from using Qigong and the population at large lost interest.

Qigong in the 20th Century

1911–1949, Republic of China

- Parallel to the ostracizing of traditional Chinese medicine, Qigong was also almost forgotten during the first two decades of the republic.
- The first attempts by several physicians to revive Qigong in modern form took place during the 1930s—first in line was Liu Guizhen.

1949 to the Present, People's Republic of China

- Traditional Chinese medicine is being restored.
- During the 1950s, traditional Chinese medicine became equal in status in China with Western medicine.
- In 1979 a National Conference on Qigong Research convened, initiated by the International Institute for traditional Chinese medicine in Beijing.
- Since the 1980s, a new euphoria has taken hold, with approximately 50 million people in China pursuing—for a greater sense of well-being or because of illness—Qigong.
- Since the late 1980s, the popularity of Qigong in the West has also continued to rise.

The Influence of Chinese Philosophy

In order to better understand the basis of Tai Chi Ch'uan and Qigong, a beginner should not only be familiar with the history of their evolution but also have some knowledge about how Tai Chi Ch'uan and Qigong are intimately related to Chinese philosophy—whose roots reach back as far as the 5th century B.C.

Practising Tai Chi Ch'uan and Qigong means more than simply being engaged in a useful exercise employing esthetically pleasing movements. Inherent to the practice is having an *inner disposition*, or frame of mind, that is based on the *philosophy of balance*, as well as the understanding that we are subject to constant changes according to the laws of nature and are becoming and passing on a cosmic process that the ancient Chinese called the Dao (also known as Tao).

The Dao

The most important characteristic of the Dao is the idea that everything in nature, in the physical world as well as in every human being, is cyclical and involves a never-ending coming and going, expansion and contraction. The cyclical pattern of the movement of the Tao is illustrated with a symbol that depicts the opposing nature of yin and yang.

However, Tai Chi Ch'uan—according to the theory of movement—consists of *acyclical* movements, where one movement flows into the next. The concept of *cyclical*, as used in philosophy, refers here first and

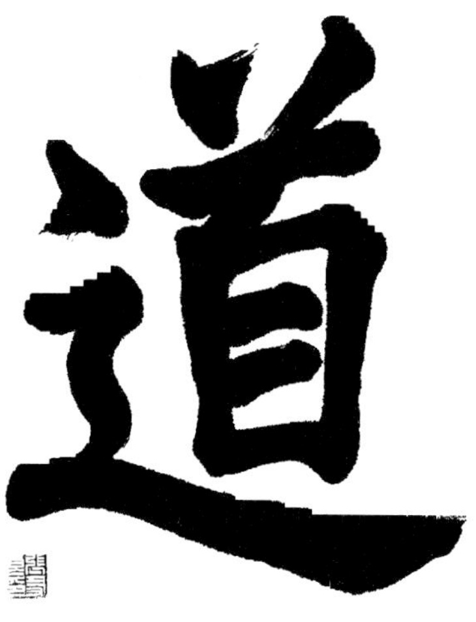

Dao or Tao

foremost to the constant change between tensing and relaxing of the musculature. So, in a sense, Tai Chi Ch'uan can be said to be both cyclical and acyclical at the same time, which only initially can be seen as a contradiction.

But to try to understand the Dao intellectually is not really all that productive. The Dao can only be fathomed through the intuition (*chin*) in a state of silence (*t'ien*), where it is felt or known.

For the ancient Chinese, Chi exercises were a means, among many others, to get to know or feel the Dao. The exercises were a way of realizing in the human body what Engelhardt has called "the intrinsic orderliness present in the cosmos." One of the fundamental principles upon which these exercises were based contends that our destiny is within us, not in the heavens.

The Yin-Yang Theory

The essence of the yin-yang theory is that everything in the world has two opposing yet complementary sides. For instance, according to the Dao, heaven is yang and the earth is yin. The heavens above are motion, the earth is calmness, and between those two poles are human beings, who, in a way, combine both of those polar energies within themselves. The upper half of the body is yang; the lower half is yin.

These energies are not static but rather dynamic, which means they all serve a purpose. Everything that moves, is active, and has strong purpose and movements belongs to yang. Everything that remains serene, is passive, and has weaker functions is yin.

The dynamic character of yin and yang is illustrated in the diagram on page 19. It consists of an

Yin & Yang Principles

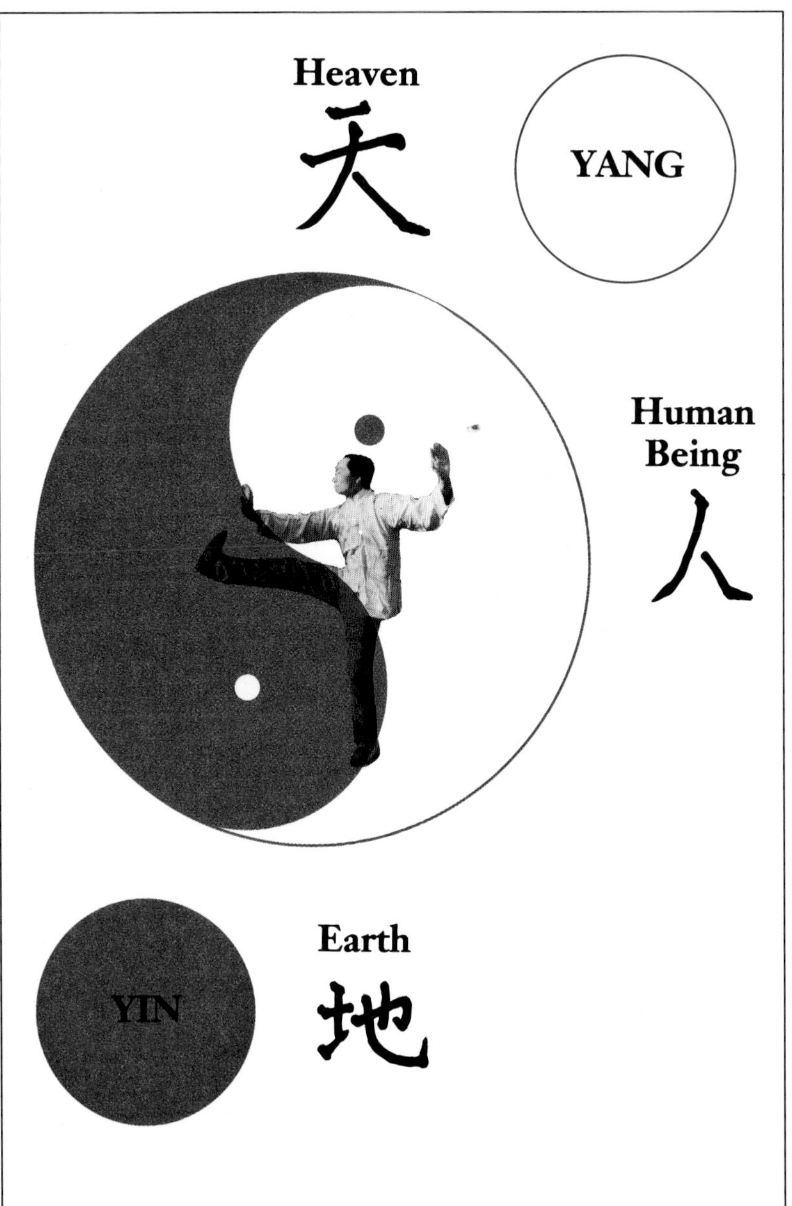

oscillating symmetry, where the dark portion represents *yin*—the earth—and the light portion *yang*—the heavens. The drawing on the previous page expresses these two energies.

Both dots in the diagram symbolize the concept that every time either of the two energies reaches an extreme position, it already carries within itself the seed of the opposite.

In the mind of the ancient Chinese, both the yin and the yang poles are not viewed as contradictory opposites but rather the different sides of the same coin.

Nothing is ever only yin or only yang. All natural phenomena

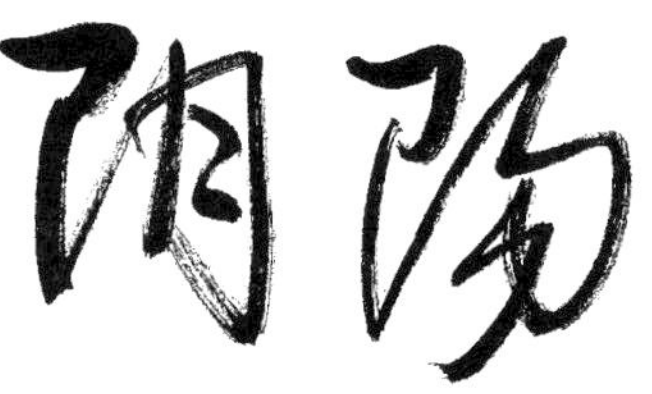

Yin and Yang

embody a continuous interplay between both poles, with all changes being fluid and following each other in unbroken succession. There is a dynamic balance between yin and yang in the natural order.

For traditional Chinese medicine and Qigong, in practical terms this means that health can only be maintained if our organisms are kept in constant movement and exchange between yin and yang.

When related to the Qigong Form that is part of the "exercises in motion," it implies practising outward motion, inner calmness, and calm movements. In such a practice, movement and calmness are rooted within each other and yin and yang are in balance.

The same principle, in general, also holds for Tai Chi Ch'uan movements. We distinguish between yin and yang movements of the arms and legs—in a constant shift between tension and relaxation. These movements are not done in isolation, but rather as a harmonious interplay—also involving the head and the body—that creates a unified whole.

In his classic text about Tai Chi Ch'uan, Wu Yuxiang states: "When one part of the body moves, the whole body is active; if a part stops moving, the whole body stops."

It can be said that, for Tai Chi Ch'uan as well as Qigong, breathing, movement, and concentration reflect an ongoing interplay between yin and yang, and that this activates the very "source" in our own body, allowing it to become one with the cosmos.

The Chi Concept

In Tai Chi Ch'uan, *Chi* is crucial and can only be understood in connection with the theory of yin and yang.

The mind directs the flow of Chi so that it can sink deeply and settle into the bones. If the Chi is flowing freely throughout the body without encountering any barriers, the mind can guide it easily. This is another principle originated by Wu Yuxiang.

What Is Chi and How Does It Work?

Is Chi a definable substance, is it matter that flows through our body, and how can it be guided or directed?

The full extent of the meaning of Chi cannot be related in just a few words. But, in general terms, the complexity of the many different meanings can be summed up as "a moment of blessing, of flow, and of expansion" (Engelhardt).

From a text written around 320 A.D., we see the all-encompassing characteristic of Chi: "Human beings are surrounded by Chi, and Chi is present in every human being."

Everything in the heavens and the natural world is in need of Chi for its very life. If we know how to guide the Chi, we are nourishing our bodies from the inside, while defending against adverse influences from the outside.

In other words, Chi not only influences our bodies, but it is present also throughout the whole of the cosmos. It affects,

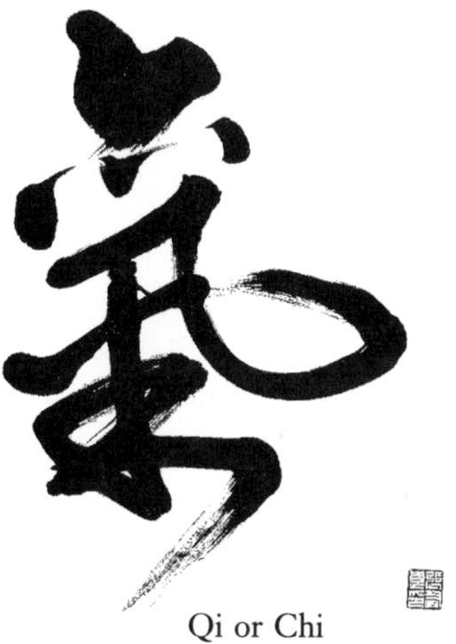

Qi or Chi

therefore, every human being from the inside as well as from the outside. In this sense, Chi could be considered part of the energy field, but it is not a measurable substance. Chi is similar to what we call energy but not the equivalent of it. Chi always seeks a qualification, or a movement pointing towards a particular direction.

The physicist F. Capra pursued the question: In what sense

could Chi be considered a form of energy as we define it in physics, which contends that energy is a quantifiable substance? Capra came to the conclusion that "Chi" does not refer to the flow of a certain substance but rather implies the principle of flow, which is always cyclical.

What is the fundamental connection between Chi and Chinese philosophy? In very simple terms, this can be said:

- Every human being has inherited a certain quality of Chi that can be very high but also very low. This inherited, or prenatal, Chi is called *Yuan Chi.*
- Chi is also given to us through food, the *Gu Chi*, or food Chi.
- The *Kong Chi* reaches our body through breathing and—together with the *Yuan Chi* and the *Gu Chi*—combines to form the overall Chi, or *Zheng Chi*, that infuses the entire body.
- *Zheng Chi* is the all-encompassing term for several types of Chi that have very specific functions.

Zheng Chi, according to traditional Chinese medicine taught at the Academy for TCM in Shanghai, has five main functions in the human body, which are summarized on page 23.

The most important function, as far as Tai Chi Ch'uan and Qigong are concerned, is that it is responsible for all movements. The quality of our Chi, however, determines our general health. In simple terms it can be said that, according to traditional Chinese medicine, the human body is a combination of yin-yang parts (meaning yin-yang organs), and a person is healthy when all these parts are in a state of harmonious balance. This balance is kept intact through an unimpeded flow of Chi (of "life energy" in the widest sense) along a system of meridians, in which the yang meridian leads to the yin organs and the yin meridian to the yang organs.

The result of a flow of Chi that is obstructed, for whatever reason, is disturbance or blockage, and the consequence is a malfunction of the respective organ; in other words, the person is sick. One method of reestablishing the flow of Chi and to heal it is by inserting needles in the respective acupuncture points that are located along the meridian.

Specific effects can be achieved from performing Chi exercises. Not only has this been shown in historic texts but in research conducted in traditional Chinese medicine.

The Chi Concept

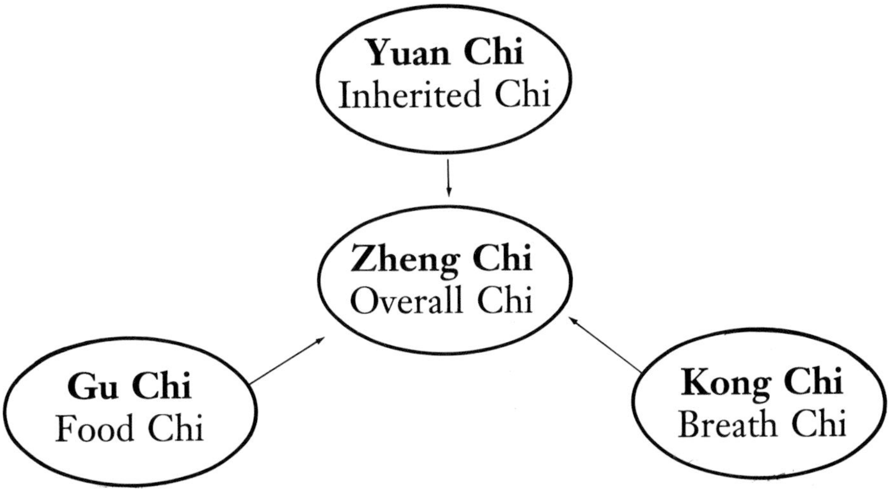

Yuan Chi
Inherited Chi

Zheng Chi
Overall Chi

Gu Chi
Food Chi

Kong Chi
Breath Chi

Functions of Chi

1. It is the source of all movements in the body, accompanying all movements.
2. It protects the body from pathological influences from the environment.
3. It is the source of the harmonious transformations in the body: (food → blood / food → urine).
4. It regulates the defense of all bodily substances and organs.
5. It keeps the body warm (regulates body temperature).

The Significance of Chi in Tai Chi Ch'uan and Qigong

Returning to the instruction given by Wu Yuxiang, the aim of Tai Chi Ch'uan is to allow the "stream of energy" to flow by means of mental guidance (Engelhardt says "by engaging the imagination") in such a way that no barriers or blockages are created. This, in turn, will preserve and strengthen the overall well-being of the person performing the exercises. Mental guidance becomes possible by correctly performing the movements according to the criteria (see pages 43–46) and principles involved in the movements. The same holds true for Qigong exercises if they are to produce maximum results.

The difference between Tai Chi Ch'uan and Qigong, as far as the physiological behavior of Chi is concerned, is that in Tai Chi Ch'uan the yang, or end phase of the form, produces Chi, meaning that it is *delivered* to the outside; while during Qigong the Chi is *taken in* by the body. For this reason alone, we can see that Tai

When father and son . . .

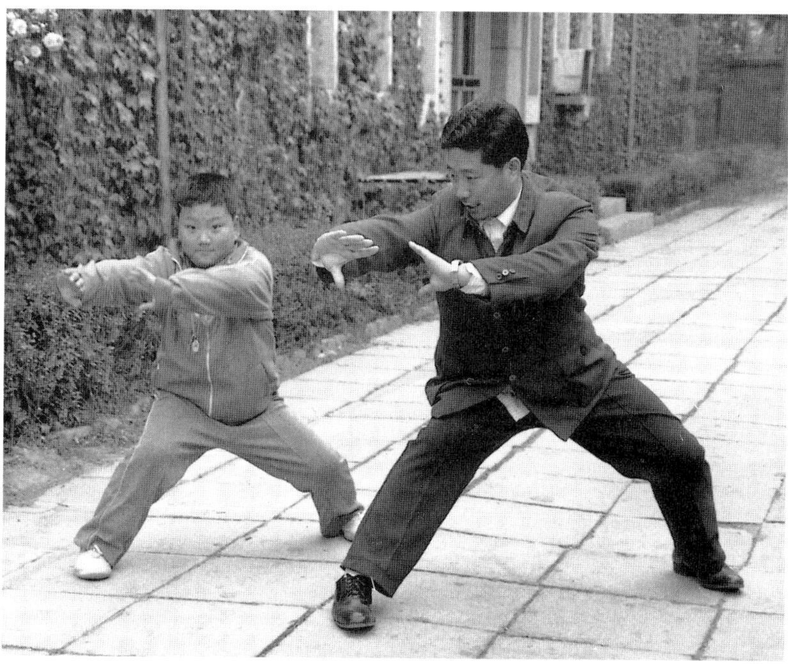

Chi Ch'uan and Qigong are an ideal complement to each other.

Using Chi

How, then, is a person to handle Chi? Don't let the complexity of the subject scare you off; rather, try first to learn the correct technique of each individual form—with much patience and perseverance. It is important to have a sense of the theory, but practising is the most important factor.

If we want to accept the Chi concept, we must be open to Chinese thinking. A discussion about the meaning of a concept such as Chi is totally foreign to the Chinese—unlike in the West, where we strive to understand everything intellectually. Neither classical nor modern Chinese texts speculate about the nature of Chi, nor do they attempt to describe it. Chi is understood in a functional framework: The Chinese are concerned with how it works.

The chief of a clinic in China was asked by a German professor for a scientific explanation of acupuncture. Though he said he would be pleased to give such an explanation, he replied that the Chinese have absolutely no interest in this question. For the Chinese, he said, it is enough that the method has worked for 2,500 years.

An Interpretation

The term *Tai Chi Ch'uan* is a combination of three characters that give expression to two concepts: Tai and Ch'uan. According to ancient Chinese thinking, the fundamental idea underlying these concepts is one of undifferentiation, which is also the fundamental basis of the world. It is, furthermore, the source of the two polar energies, yin and yang, which, through their reciprocal interaction, brought the world into being. The concept of *Tai* appears for the first time in the *Book of Changes* (*I Ching*), where it says that *Tai Chi* is contained in change, which brings forth the two energies, yin and yang.

The concept of *Ch'uan* can be defined in three different ways:

1 Fighting with empty fists (fighting without a weapon)

2 Collecting life's energies internally

3 Balance between both yin and yang energies

Chen Xin, one of the spokesmen of the Chen school, was the first to use Tai Chi Ch'uan as a collective term. In his book, *Tai Chi Ch'uan*, Chen states: "The term *Ch'uan* also means balance;

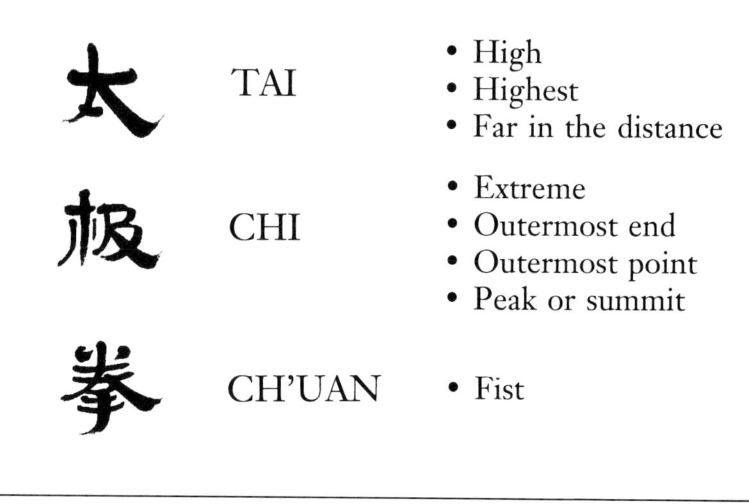

太
TAI
• High
• Highest
• Far in the distance
极
CHI
• Extreme
• Outermost end
• Outermost point
• Peak or summit
拳
CH'UAN
• Fist

What Is Tai Chi Ch'uan?

that is why one weighs things in order to determine their significance. But the fundamental principle [of Tai Chi Ch'uan] is rooted in the reality of *Tai*, and this means that its application is inseparably connected to the fists. In addition, the whole human body—from head to toe—represents Tai, while it is—at the same time—Ch'uan. Ch'uan should not only be seen as merely representing fists."

Tai Chi Ch'uan Summary

Tai Chi Ch'uan, as defined by the Chinese, implies creating a connection to one's origin-of-being through practice with the fists (Ch'uan). Also implied is observing the law of yin and yang in order to be part of the universal energies of nature and thus coming into balance with the universe. The highest and ultimate goal is to achieve, to the greatest extent possible, harmony and balance by observing the order in nature.

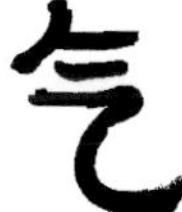

QI (CHI)

- Steam
- Smoke
- Breath
- Life energy

功 GONG (KUNG)

- Success
- Performance
- Effect

What Is Qigong (Chi Kung)?

An Interpretation

The term *Qigong* is also a combination of two concepts, *Qi* (or *Chi*) *Gong* (or *Kung*). *Gong* is often translated as "work" and, in combination with *Qi*, as "to work with Chi." Yet we believe that that does not take the full meaning into account. People often say that Qigong (and Tai Chi Ch'uan) can't really be translated at all, and we tend to agree, although we would like to offer the beginner at least a general definition.

Qigong Summary

For the Chinese, practising *Qigong* means to bring, through specific energy-supporting breathing exercises, the Chi that flows through the human body into harmony with the Chi that permeates the cosmos. Here, too, the highest goal is to reach and protect our spiritual well-being.

2
Tai Chi Ch'uan & Qigong: Antidote to Today's Stress

Stress & Time

To the question "What is stress?," most people would respond the way the church father Augustine did: "*Quid est tempus?*" ['What is time?']: "If nobody asks, I will know. But if I begin to explain it to somebody who has asked, then I won't know."

Science, as well, to this day, has been unable to give a final and definitive explanation. This is understandable if we take into consideration that human beings have their own individual perceptions of the world and may react very differently to one and the same situation. What is stressful for one person is not necessarily stressful for another. Furthermore, according to scientific findings, our genetic makeup has been increasingly seen to play a role in stress-related illnesses. In addition, medical experts have found that a prolonged rise in the level of adrenaline and cortisone—due to stress—leads to damage of the heart and circulatory system and to the reduction in functioning of the nerve cells that are important for short-term memory. But how much is too much for any given individual, essentially, must be determined by that individual.

Nevertheless, surely one of the most destructive stresses has to do with the lack of time. This is a stress many of us encounter daily.

- At work: deadlines, performance pressure
- At home: problems in balancing career and family
- Free time: social obligations, other activities

Are we human beings helpless in the face of the furious tempo of today's society? Can we do anything about it?

Slowing Down vs. Rushing

What we lose when we gain time is illustrated in the following story: A very old, devout Muslim was preparing for a pilgrimage to Mecca. After much prodding from his family, he decided against making the trip by foot, a burdensome undertaking, and took a plane instead. On his return, he was asked how it was. The old man replied that his spirit did not seem to have been in Mecca at all, because, he said, "The spirit walks."

To remain untouched by the hectic pace of modern times is virtually impossible for most of us. What is possible, however, is that we, as human beings, unlike the members of the animal world, can analyze our situation and make changes. And it is precisely for this reason that a specific stress need not remain a stress. We have it in our power to influence the rhythm of our life, which means that in many situations we can *slow down.* This could begin, very simply, at the breakfast table in the way we chew our food and in how we decide to relax before retiring at night.

Tai Chi Ch'uan & Qigong as Slowing-Down Exercises

Practising Tai Chi Ch'uan and Qigong makes it possible to slow down the pace of our life. Yang Chengfu (mentioned earlier), one of the founding fathers of Tai Chi Ch'uan, said in *The 10 Basic Principles of Tai Chi Ch'uan:* "In Tai Chi Ch'uan, movements are born in peacefulness; even when in motion, all remains calm. That is why the movements of a form should be performed as slowly as possible."

The Buddhist monk and teacher Nyanaponika Mahathera in *Mental Training Through Attentiveness* said: "To counter the unhealthy effects of the frantic pace of modern life, it is imperative that, in our free time, we try consciously to pause and slow down. . . . Slowing down is helpful in reducing mental and physical tension. . . . Beyond the immediate effects of an exercise session, slowing-down exercises influence the pace of the daily rhythm in what we do, how we talk and think."

Tai Chi Ch'uan & Medicine

Medical Benefits in General

For millions of Chinese people, Tai Chi Ch'uan is practised on a daily basis, either of their own volition or prescribed as therapy in hospitals and sanatoriums.

What makes Tai Chi Ch'uan so valuable, and what are the effects on the health and overall well-being of a person?

We do not intend to repeat here the many accounts found in other books about the illnesses and complaints that have been positively affected through the practice of Tai Chi Ch'uan. However, every beginner will observe that Tai Chi Ch'uan fully mobilizes the whole body, the active as well as the passive parts. The leg muscles, in particular, are challenged and strengthened, because they continuously alternate between tensing and relaxing. This makes Tai Chi Ch'uan an ideal exercise for skiers. As a load-bearing activity, with the legs carrying the body, Tai Chi Ch'uan is also a terrific means of supporting an increase in bone mass, making it an ideal exercise to counteract osteoporosis.

Tai Chi Ch'uan is also excellent for addressing flexibility, because of the gentle way that movements are carried out, preserving and improving mobility of the joints and stretching the muscles.

Benefits for the Heart and Circulatory System and the Metabolism—Scientific Research in China

We are referring to research conducted at the Wushu Research Institute in Beijing, which was published at the convention of the International Wushu Festival in 1988. The background for this research is as follows: There are several universities and colleges on the western outskirts of Beijing where more than 40,000 people work as teachers, consultants, and administrators. A survey regarding the state of their health was conducted in the 1970s and the beginning of the 1980s, and the results were alarming. The life expectancy of the university and college teachers was 58—10 years less than that of the general population. The primary cause of death was illnesses of the heart and circulatory system, due to:

- Improper nutrition and being overweight
- Stress
- Sedentary lifestyles

Consequently, the following countermeasures were taken: In 1975 the Tai Chi Ch'uan Guidance Club was started to promote and foster health, and 10 years later, in 1985, the Wushu Association of the Chinese Academy was founded under the leadership of experts in the field. As a result of these two programs, at least 20,000 individuals are actively taking part and regularly attending Tai Chi Ch'uan classes! For this research, which continued from 1983 to 1986, the following indicators were used.

EEG (Electroencephalogram)

Bioelectrical activities of nerve cells change when the organism is under psychological stress, when sense organs are active, and during illness. With the help of an electroencephalograph—electrodes attached to different places on the head—the activities of the brain are recorded. Science distinguishes mainly between alpha, beta, and theta waves, all of which are said to be influenced by specific, subjective sensations.

EKG (Electrocardiogram)

The EKG measures changes in electrical tension that are spread over the entire body and registered on the surface of the skin. This procedure is helpful in the diagnosis of irregularities in the rhythm of the heart and of other heart problems.

Measuring Blood Lipids (Serum Lipids)

The level of serum lipids is determined by examining a blood sample. Comparing the data to preestablished norms, the level of serum lipids is either normal or dangerous to the health of the individual. A significant elevation above the norm (hyperlipema) almost always means that the individual is in danger of suffering heart problems and blood vessel diseases, including those of the brain.

Testing

The subjects, whose average age was 50, were divided into two groups. One group consisted of men and women who had practised Tai Chi Ch'uan for five years or more (five to seven times per week). This group was given the name Tai Chi Ch'uan Group. The other group was made up of men and women who had not been involved in any kind of athletic activity or had only been practising Tai Chi Ch'uan for a couple of weeks. This was the control group.

Twenty to 30 people in each group underwent EEG and EKG examinations. Serum lipids examinations were conducted on a total of more than 100 people. Each of the EEG and EKG examinations were done before and after a 30-minute exercise period. The EEG and EKG measurements were taken twice: once before exercising, with the individuals lying down, and again within 5 minutes after the exercises were completed. Pulse and breathing frequency were also measured.

For the test results, the researcher chose the Beijing Short Form and the 48 Forms, which consist of several different sequences; the latter is still the most popular form in China, and the one that can be observed most frequently in parks.

Results and Conclusions

The Tai Chi Ch'uan Group showed a marked increase in alpha-wave activity. When questioned as to how they felt, participants stated that they felt *balanced, relaxed, mentally alert* and *focused*.

The participants in the control group, on the other hand, showed little change in alpha-wave activity; only in a few instances was there a slight increase in alpha waves and a slight decrease in beta waves.

EKG Measurements The Tai Chi Ch'uan Group registered an increase in the blood volume of the heart muscle and a positive influence on the regulation of the heart rates in cases of tachycardia (increased heart rate) and bradycardia (very slow heart rate). Participants with coronary blood vessel problems did exercises adjusted for their condition and showed improvements.

Because Tai Chi Ch'uan movements are slow and gentle, individuals are always in control of how intense they want an exercise to be. Damage to the heart, therefore, is nearly impossible.

Thus, Tai Chi Ch'uan is almost an ideal exercise for heart patients.

Effects on Serum Lipids The target value of the serum lipids (cholesterol, beta lipoprotein, and triglycerides) was either not at all, or only slightly higher, in the Tai Chi Ch'uan Group.

For individuals who had been exercising for a long period of time, the explanation for this is as follows: The brain of an individual during exercise and for some time after is in a significant state of alertness (primarily revealed in alpha-wave activity), and the person is calm and relaxed. This overall state is helpful in reducing or lessening symptoms of pathological stress. It, furthermore, influences the concentration of corticosteroids (adrenal) hormones in the blood and allows the level of adrenaline in the blood to remain normal. As a result, the level of serum lipids is reduced, slowing down the deposits of LDLs (low-density lipoproteins) on the walls of the arteries, which can lead to arteriosclerosis.

In addition, breathing deeply from the belly—a requirement when doing Tai Chi Ch'uan—strengthens the diaphragm, resulting in an increased massage like action of the liver, which, in turn, influences the metabolic process and lowers the level of serum lipids.

Influence on Heart Rate and Oxygen Uptake—A Japanese Study

The following material was taken from a study, written in 1992 by K. Matsui, P. Zhou, and K. Suguyama of the Department of Physical Education at Shizuoka University in Japan, with the title *On the Changing Heart Rate During Tai Chi Ch'uan Performance by an Expert.*

Goal of the Study

The team wanted to determine the load intensity of different Tai Chi Ch'uan styles in relation to *heart rate* and *maximum oxygen uptake* and to compare the two. We were interested in the results obtained from exercises in the Beijing Short Form, presented in this book.

The Protocol

Peifang Zhou (a coauthor of this book) was a participant in this study and, at the time, 37 years old and a runner-up in the Yang Tai Chi Ch'uan Championships in China.

First, the researcher established a maximum load test with the help of a bicycle spiro-ergometer, while simultaneously performing an EKG. The bicycle spiro-ergometer measured the vital capacity (the maximum volume exhaled after maximum air has been inhaled), and the resulting value, accounting for statistical deviation, was converted to maximum oxygen intake per minute. The EKG measured the heart rate under maximum load.

During the experiment, a portable telemetric pulse-measuring device recorded the heart rate in 10-second intervals, which were then prorated into one-minute readings. Measurements were also taken and recorded 10 seconds before and after the exercise. During the measurements, the extent of the knee bends also played a vital role, as that determined the load intensity during each stage and, thus, the influence on heart rate and oxygen consumption. For this reason, the experimenter distinguished between slight, medium, and deep bends. Of course, it is important to note that the degree to which knees are bent is always a subjective determination. The three different levels of difficulty have one thing in common: The heart-rate frequency increases by 10 beats in the last third of each of the three levels (the same holds for oxygen consumption) and returns to normal towards the end.

The increase is due to the most difficult part of the sequence: two "dropped-whip" sequences following each other.

Chart 1. Load Intensity in Relation to Knee Bends

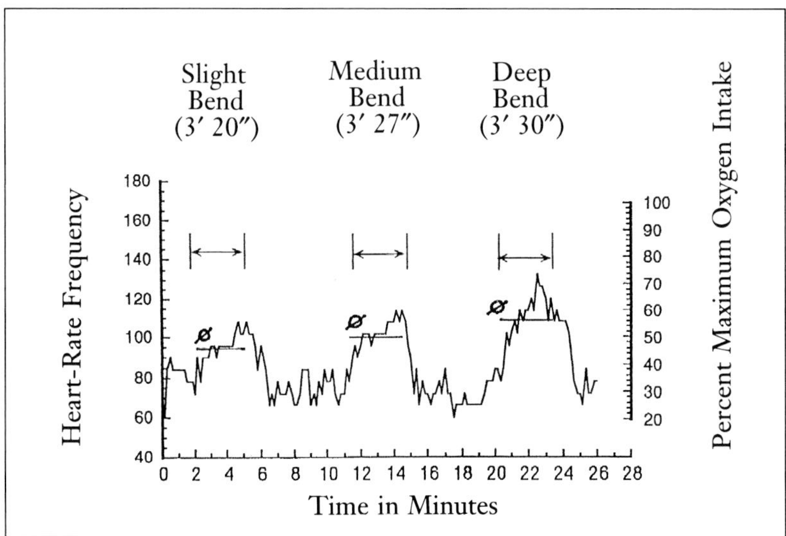

The load intensity of the Beijing Short Form is shown here. The Form was performed three times with a rest period between each.

Slight Bends: The average heart-rate frequency remained below 100/minute, with a maximum oxygen intake of about 72%.

Deep Bends: Here, the heart rate increased to 120/minute about 2 minutes after the measurement began. Oxygen intake was about 65%; later, the values increased to 132/minute and 72%, respectively.

Results and Conclusions

When the results were analyzed, we realized that by using a well-trained athlete in Tai Chi Ch'uan, the results would only be meaningful if we took into account the fitness level of the average person. However, as Chart 4 on the next page clearly shows, the Short Beijing Form can easily be adjusted to any individual's age and physical condition. Thus, for a person at an average fitness level, a heart rate of about 130/minute can be achieved,

Chart 2. Slight Bend—Performed Three Times in a Row

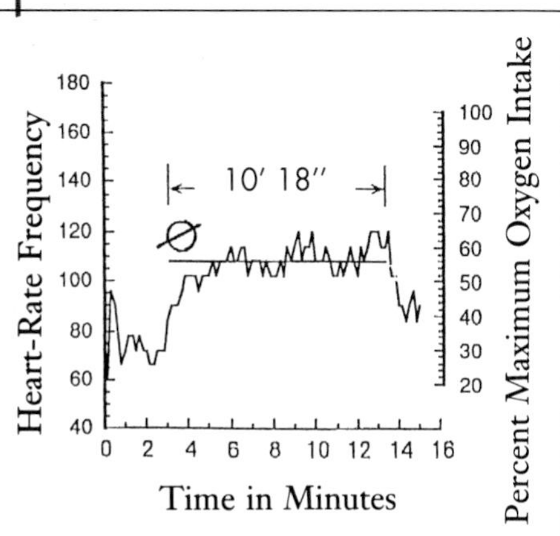

Chart 3. Deep Bend—Performed Three Times in a Row

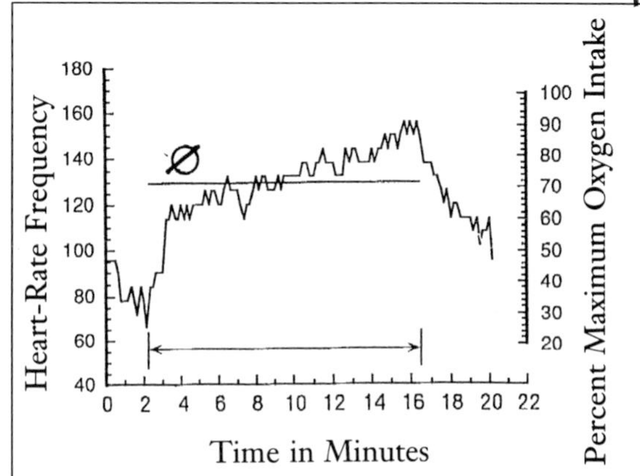

These charts show the different load intensity during three performances of the Beijing Short Form that followed each other without a rest in between.

Slight Bend (Chart 2): The heart rate already is increasing during the second stage to a maximum value of 120/minute, the same rate reached in the third stage but without further increase.

Deep Bend (Chart 3): The heart rate has already increased to 120/minute (about 65% of normal oxygen intake) 2 minutes after recording the measurement began; during the following 12 minutes, it reached a maximum value of 155/minute (about 85% of the maximum oxygen intake).

Load-Bearing Capacity during Tai Chi Ch'uan (Beijing Short Form)	Duration	Maximum Heart Rate	Medium Heart Rate (with standard deviation)	Medium Percent Maximum Oxygen Intake (with standard deviation)
Slight Bend	3.20	108	94.9 ± 8.6	45.2 ± 6.3
Medium Bend	3.27	114	99.0 ± 10.8	48.1 ± 7.9
Deep Bend	3.30	132	107.5 ± 14.9	54.4 ± 11.0
Slight Bend (three in a row)	10.17	120	106.9 ± 7.6	53.9 ± 5.7
Deep Bend (three in a row)	14.10	156	129.7 ± 15.3	70.7 ± 11.2

Chart 4. Summary of Charts 1–3

which represents an ideal goal for cardiovascular training, when the aim is to improve stamina, comparable to that of a reasonable jogging, bicycling, or swimming regimen.

The average oxygen intake will be around 60 percent, which represents a medium and very pleasant load intensity and won't cause overexertion.

Conclusions

1. The positive effects on muscles, bones, and joints when practising Tai Chi Ch'uan are undisputed.

2. The studies conducted at the Wushu Research Institute and at Shizuoka University show that Tai Chi Ch'uan can be used as a means of preventing and treating illnesses that involve the heart and circulatory system, brain function, and metabolism. Tai Chi Ch'uan was also found to be ideal for aerobic fitness training, because it can be undertaken without any danger to one's health—particularly for middle-aged and older people.

3. What distinguishes Tai Chi Ch'uan from most other fitness programs is the psychological and physiological aspects that are clearly demonstrated by the EEG test results: the phenomena of the alpha wave, indicating that the organism is in a state of wakefulness and is completely relaxed. We can only produce alpha waves when we have eliminated all thought and, therefore, freed ourselves of worries. Thus, practising Tai Chi Ch'uan is an ideal means of entering into a resting phase devoid of any stress.

Qigong & Medicine

General Medical Benefits

Qigong exercises are a means of supporting the treatment of illnesses. Prevention of illnesses and treatment of chronic disorders are the main reasons for recommending Qigong. What are the effects of this type of exercise? Jiao Guorui, the director of the Institute for Qigong at the Academy for Traditional Chinese Medicine in Beijing, explained that the primary reason for doing Qigong exercises has to do with the training of the Chi, in order to keep the biological processes moving in the human organism—which is in a very intimate relationship with the environment.

Internal activity within the body is ongoing in all organs, functional systems, and metabolic processes. Breathing, digestion, blood circulation—all physiological as well as psychological activities—are different and dynamic internal processes. These processes, involved with taking away the old and replacing it with the new, can only be healthy and fluid with the transformation of the Chi. The effectiveness of Qigong has to do with the fact that it strengthens the transformation of the Chi through posture, breathing, and the power of the imagination.

In the early 1960s, a medical researcher in Shanghai studying the effects of Qigong discovered that the heart rate, breathing frequency, and oxygen consumption of subjects began to slow down considerably during the resting phase, perhaps as a result of the accumulation of energy. In the late 1970s, a Chinese scientist at the Nuclear Research Institute at the Academy for Science found that physiological changes were taking place during Qigong exercises, including an increase in the activity of the gallbladder and a lowering of blood pressure.

Specific Effects

Experimental research, clinical applications, and geriatric medicine in China all confirm that Qigong exercises—in conjunction with other therapies (including, for instance, Western drug treatment)—shorten recovery time and strengthen treatment results. This was observed in illnesses including bronchial asthma, tuberculosis, stomach and small intestinal ulcers, and disorders of the heart and nervous system.

It's also important to note that, during Qigong exercises, the alpha waves show definite changes, pointing to a heightened state of relaxation. This is similar to what happens when performing Tai Chi Ch'uan.

Summary

In general, it can be stated that Qigong, if practised on a regular basis, regulates the autonomic system—meaning that it positively influences breathing, digestion, the heart and the circulatory system, oxygen exchange, and the nervous system. By concentrating on breathing and on the movement of particular parts of the body, Qigong is able to dissolve tension, to gently mobilize the body through movement, and to contribute in a very comfortable way to an overall state of well-being.

Choosing the Beijing Short Form

As mentioned earlier, the Beijing Short Form is based on the Yang style. This Form was developed by experts from China's National Sports Commission in 1956. It consists of a sequence of 24 consecutive forms (after 1956, sequences of 48 and 88 forms were added). Each sequence has it own name. Some forms also include offensive or defensive movements, but they are combined into a whole.

These forms are not just simple movements, but rather a meaningful collection of original sequences that sometimes have included more than 80—sometimes even more than 100—forms, where more than a third are repetitions.

Performing the Beijing Short Form takes about 3½ to 4½ minutes.

The historical evolution of Tai Chi Ch'uan has shown that, during the formation of individual schools, constant changes, corrections, and innovations took place. Particularly in recent decades, as a result of new findings in the area of biomechanics, aspects of Tai Chi Ch'uan that were thoroughly studied have been improved.

The Beijing Short Form is ideal for the beginner, particularly because of the:

- sound structure of the sequences,
- easy comprehension of the sequences,
- thoughtful attention to the increase in the degree of difficulty, and
- suitable number of forms—making for a manageable exercise program.

Criteria for Performing Tai Chi Ch'uan Movements

When learning Tai Chi Ch'uan, beginners are often confronted with too many details, which may make them reluctant to continue—or even want to abandon it altogether. For this reason, we will deal with the essential criteria for movements first and then discuss the mental components. These criteria are slow, easy, round (or circular). They also have continuity, differentiation between empty and full, and are harmonious.

Slow

In the Beijing Short Form, movements throughout are performed equally slowly and quietly. The total form should take about 4 minutes, on the average. Because of the low, flowing movements, the body can relax and become calm, and external tranquility becomes internal. If a person becomes centered, this tranquility is projected outward again.

The slow movements allow a

person to concentrate on the details and mentally prepare for the next movement.

Easy

"Easy" in Tai Chi Ch'uan means avoiding unnecessary use of energy and muscle tension and carrying out all movements sensibly and economically. Among other criteria, well-coordinated movements are recognized by the way they reach their target and their economy and ease.

The Chinese often compare the ease of these exercises to the way clouds seem to move weightlessly in the sky.

Round

All movements in Tai Chi Ch'uan are either round (or circular) or arched. As discussed earlier, Tai Chi Ch'uan grew out of offensive and defensive techniques. Circular movements hide from an opponent the starting point as well the exact target of a movement. If the opponent reacts offensively by "hitting" a circle, the energy will be deflected tangentially off the circle. Consequently, round movements are very advantageous if you want to trick an opponent or defend yourself.

In Tai Chi Ch'uan, the flow of the movements is determined by their circular quality. Every change in direction of a movement will demonstrate an optimum flow if it is round or arched.

Continuity

Every movement within a form is performed in one *continuous* flow. In other words, individual movements are connected in flowing motion—without breaking or jerking—in space, time, or dynamics. Optimum flow is present when internal and external energies are aligned as much as possible.

Differentiation Between Empty and Full

This is a difficult subject, and we will try to explain it as simply as possible without misrepresenting the principles of Tai Chi Ch'uan that have been handed down to us. *Empty* and *full*, if understood as synonymous with "neutral" and "weightiness," refer to the interrelatedness of *yin* and *yang* movements. Yin is considered to be emptiness or neutrality, and yang fullness or weightiness. But *empty*—for instance—does not mean that a foot is totally uninvolved (does not carry any weight); nor does *full* mean that a foot carries the full weight of the body. In the forward, arched step in the end phase—for instance—the proportion of the weight distribution between both feet is expressed in a ratio of about 70:30.

In somewhat simplified terms, one could say that any expanding—forward or upward—movement is yang and any contracting movement—pulling back or down—is yin.

As the Yin & Yang Principles diagram on page 19 demonstrates quite clearly, at the moment of greatest expansion of the yang portion, the essence of yin is already present. The same holds true for the yin portion in relation to yang.

The succession of yin and yang phases creates a rhythmical interplay whose poles are characterized as tension (yang) and relaxation (yin). To put it another way, both phases bring about a very specific rhythm to every movement.

Rhythmically alternating between tension and relaxation indicates a continuous exchange between putting forth and receiving of energy. According to traditional Chinese thinking, *Chi*, or energy, is constantly being exchanged between a person and the cosmos. Without this exchange, our bodies would soon tire and—eventually—be unable to move at all.

Harmonious

In Tai Chi Ch'uan, it can be said that individual movements are *harmonious* when they are coordinated to such an extent that the exercise becomes a whole. This requires the best possible coordination of all round movements of the body and the extremities. Harmony also takes place when there is a concurrence between intended, felt, and experienced movements with their actual performance.

However, in order to achieve the greatest possible harmony, it is not enough to have the necessary physical components in place; rather, a person must also be willing, from an internal standpoint, to explore and incorporate the very essence of Tai Chi Ch'uan. And what is this essence? It has to do with the ability to stay in one's own center of gravity—physically, mentally, and psychologically—and the awareness and protection of one's center.

A Word about Breathing

Proper breathing in Tai Chi Ch'uan—meaning to inhale and exhale at the right moment—plays a very important role and should never be neglected. Beginners, however, have their hands full learning the intricate sequences of a form and the criteria for movements, so that an additional concentration on breathing could be more of a hindrance at this time. This is why teachers in China—when teaching beginning students—do not pay too much attention to the breathing but allow the students to breathe normally. Later, when the students have learned the rough form, they should try to breathe from deep within, which means to breathe from the belly or the diaphragm.

The basic guidelines for inhaling and exhaling can generally be said to be the following:

- When pulling back, inhale.
- When going forward, exhale.
- When reaching up, inhale.
- When reaching down, exhale.

Beginning students should keep these "rules" in mind but first give their full attention to learning the individual forms.

Mental Aspect of Practising Tai Chi Ch'uan

Zhang Sanfeng, Wang Zongye, Wu Yuxiang, Yang Chengfu—all authors of so-called classical writings—constantly emphasized in Tai Chi Ch'uan the superiority of the spirit over the body.

- First the mind, then the body.
- First use the mind, then muscle power.
- All concentration should be on the mind and not on breathing.
- Find stillness in your movements.

These propositions do nothing less than emphasize the importance of putting one's full concentration on performing the exercises, so that every form within a sequence is executed to the best of one's ability.

A modern interpretation of what the old Tai Chi Ch'uan masters called for is bringing an attitude of automatic, relaxed, focused attention to the process.

In practical terms, this means, at the beginning of the exercise, in an upright position, to take a moment to quiet yourself and to concentrate on relaxing all muscles—facial, neck, shoulder, arm, hip, and leg. It means accepting, without resistance or judgment, your surroundings, the thoughts in your head, and your emotions, while at the same time mentally preparing for the movements that you are about to perform.

During the exercises make sure that your eyes always look in the direction of the goal; for instance, the eyes follow the hand that is performing the *hit*, *push*, or *pull*. Of course, the eyes are not fixed rigidly on the leading hand, but also take the surroundings into account.

3
Tai Chi Ch'uan & Principles of Athletic Movements

Basic Elements of Athletic Movements

This chapter discusses the basic elements that make up and are used to describe athletic movements in general.

We trust that this discussion will make it easier for you to comprehend the, sometimes difficult, movements involved in Tai Chi Ch'uan. All athletic movements can be categorized from the following perspectives:

- **The Spatial/Time Perspective** This has to do with the separation of movements into different stages that, relevant to the task and the overall objective, fulfill different functions and are interrelated.
- **The Functional/Anatomical Perspective** Of interest here are the questions of what group of muscles is involved and in which position of a movement, and of what type of muscle contractions is involved.
- **The Dynamics of the Process** This entails the intensity of the energy used and the impulses transferred from one part of the body to another, as well as

Space and Time Sequence in a Golf Swing

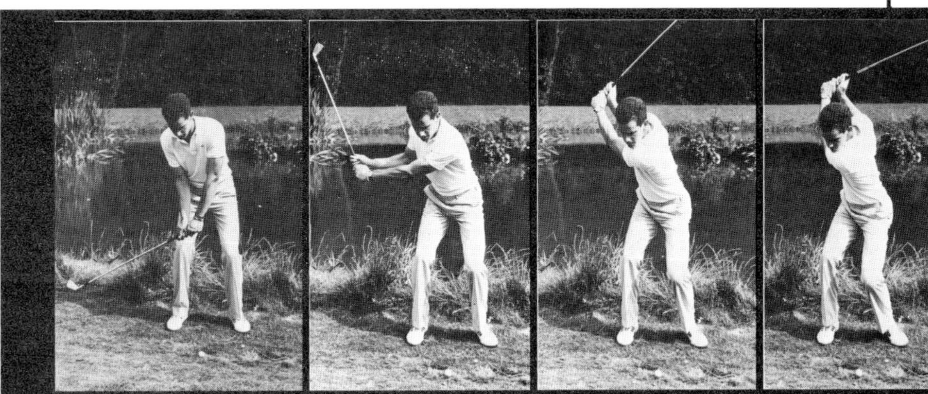

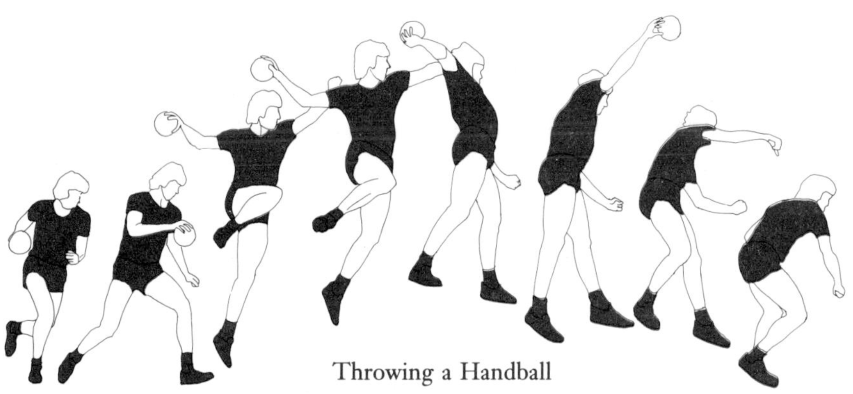
Throwing a Handball

the coordination of internal and external energies (today, such knowledge is obtained through biomechanical measuring devices).

• **The Internal Processes of Guiding and Controlling**
These can be realized from the knowledge gained from practice and theoretical information.

What follows are examples of athletic movements, presented in simplified form, that touch on some aspects discussed above. They will allow us to better understand the movements involved in Tai Chi Ch'uan. If we look at the sequence of movements performed by golfers and handball players, we will be able to distinguish between the different elements of the *spatial/time* aspect.

1. In both sports, the player starts the movement in the opposite direction from the intended

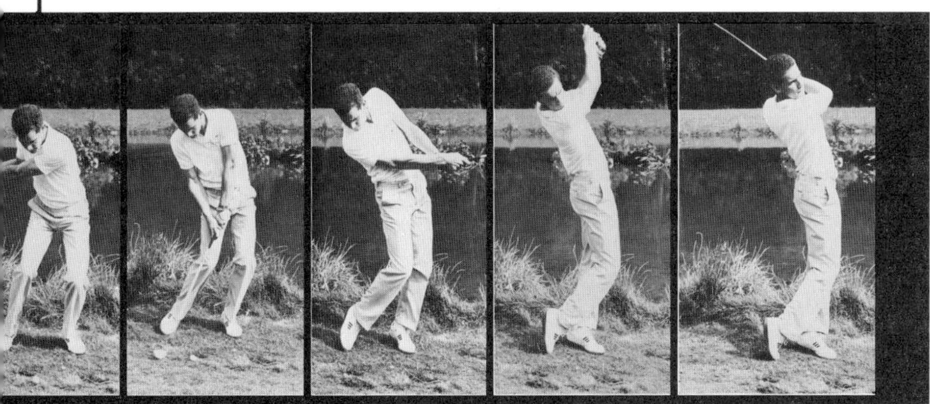

goal: the **backswing** (athletes call it the "preparation phase").

2. Next comes the **main phase,** in which the actual hit (golf) or throw (handball) takes place.

3. The **end phase** obviously follows, starting, in our example, after the golf club has hit the ball or, in handball, after the player has thrown the ball and regained balance.

The sequence of these cyclical movements (single movements, as in throwing, hitting, and Tai Chi Ch'uan) always occurs in that order and cannot be reversed.

The individual stages characterized in the Summary of Golf Swing or Handball Throw (page 47) are closely related to each other, and their dynamic pattern is executed without a break; this is very important, because, otherwise, the energy created to reach the goal would be depleted. Let us now look at additional details of this process.

The Functional Relationships

(See Summary of Golf Swing or Handball Throw on page 47.)

• The success of each individual phase depends on the result of the one preceding it (relationship to the end result).

• In the process of preparing for the next phase, the backswing (in the case of golf) is already secondary in importance to all actions of the main phase—the downswing—and the downswing, in turn, is secondary to the follow-through (causal relationship).

• The main phase (downswing) is always followed by the end phase (follow-through) (causal relationship); however, a backswing does not necessarily have to be followed by the main phase (downswing), because a player might decide to stop and not proceed to the main phase.

The Dynamics of the Process

• As far as generating the momentum of energy is concerned, the backswing and downswing must be regarded as one unit, because the energy of breaking the backward movement at the end of the backswing (where direction is reversed) must go directly into the main phase/downswing; in actual situations where the necessary speed of the movement is important, no hesitation should occur. This moment of changing direction is just about the most important stage in all athletic movements.

Summary of Golf Swing or Handball Throw

Preparation Phase or Backswing (P)	Main Phase (M)	End Phase (E)
1. The purpose of P is to create an ideal situation for M. **2.** This means creating a favorable situation for the muscles to work and the joints to bend, and to be aware of the body's correct center of gravity. **3.** At the end of P, the movement stops, which increases the tension in the musculature. This tension, at the moment the direction is reversed, is transferred to the speed of M. **4.** P can consist of several parts, such as approach run, approach slide, or approach swing, which move in the direction of M; however, the final part of P always moves in the opposite direction. Observe, for example, handball—moving the throwing arm back—and golf—swinging the club back and anchoring the right leg on the ground.	**1.** The purpose of is to create the actual forward movement by . . . **2.** This means making use of the optimal internal and external energies and optimal coordination of the impulses. **3.** Theoretically, M begins when the impulse is given for the movement. In handball, this is when the body and the throwing arm arch back. In golf, the tension created by rotating or twisting the right leg, trunk, and shoulder and the arching of the whole body is carried to the arms and the golf club.	**1.** The purpose is to actively stop the forward movement and to regain stable or dynamic balance. **2.** It is also to create a favorable center of gravity and to prepare the musculature for the acyclical movements that are to follow.

Relationship of the Three Phases of Athletic Movement

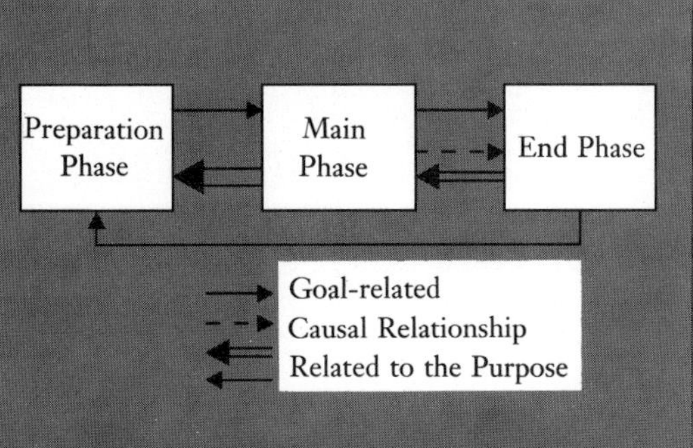

Form 4 Brushing Your Knees & Stepping

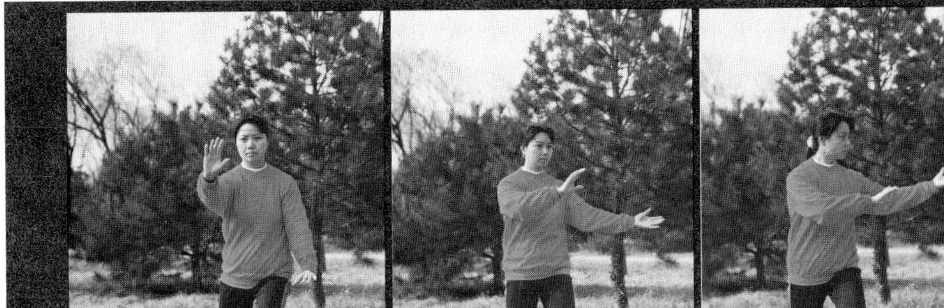

1 2 3

• It is important for the player to understand which muscles are involved or know about the energy that is required at the moment the direction is reversed. In addition, the player should have the conviction that he or she is able to coordinate all partial movements, because, on the basis of the physiology involved and according to biomechanical principles, every change in the movement of one part of the body affects all parts adjacent to it.

Every athletic movement involves the total body, even if muscles of some parts of the body are not actively engaged in the movement. Certain movements call on different parts of the body—like the legs, trunk, arms, and head—yet it's important to realize that a movement is not the sum of its parts, but always a complete entity.

Combining Several Acyclical Movements

• If several acyclical movements are carried out in succession (as in gymnastics and Tai Chi Ch'uan), there is usually a blending together of different phases, for instance, between the end phase and the previous movement and the preparation phase of the movement that follows. This is called a combination of movements.

• When movements are combined, several elements need to

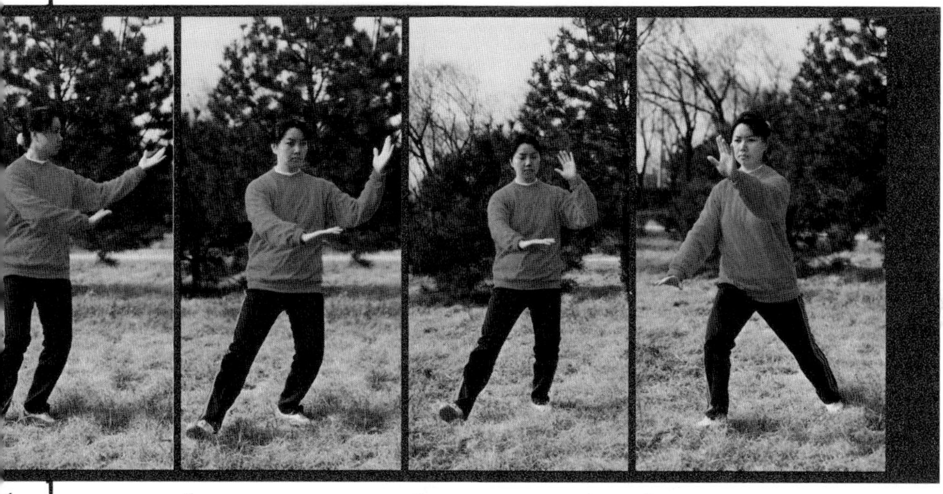

4 5 6 7

come into play: a timely engagement of the musculature and the optimal use of energy, the coordination of partial movements, and—in particular—a kinesthetic sense for the movements.

What follows is a more detailed discussion, using Tai Chi Ch'uan movements as an example.

Phases of Movements within Tai Chi Ch'uan

What we have just said about the principles of movement in general can easily be understood within the context of Tai Chi Ch'uan.

Single Movement from Form 4 Brushing Your Knees & Stepping

Form 4 Brushing Your Knees & Stepping consists of three acyclical movements that are mirror images and performed consecutively. The series of photos above illustrate one of the three movements that are part of the total of Form 4; it is a combination of acyclical movements.

In the **first photo,** we see the end phase of the first sequence, while already beginning the **preparation/backswing** (an acyclical movement).

The **backswing phase** starts out in the opposite direction of the main phase, up to the point where the weight is shifted fully to the right leg (**second photo**), so that, from that point on, the center of gravity can be shifted smoothly to the left leg (see **photos 3 and 4**).

After the weight shifting is completed, the muscle tension in the left leg increases due to the pressure of the foot on the ground, a pressure that is released at the lowest point of the knee bend (reversing direction from the backswing phase to the main phase), which is the beginning of the **main/downswing phase,** as shown in **photos 5–7.** The way the main phase is carried out is similar to the technique used in self-defense: The right hand pulls back in defense, while the left hand simultaneously goes on the offensive with a forward motion.

The position in **photo 7** represents the **end phase/follow-through,** where the sequence of movements is concluded on the left side.

Shifting the weight alternately from the right to the left knee during the course of the sequence makes optimal use of internal and external energies as well as perfectly coordinating the partial impulses—specifically, the transfer of movement impulses from the legs to the muscles of the back and to the shoulders and arms.

In a classic text said to have been written by one of the legendary founders of Tai Chi Ch'uan, Chan Sanfeng, and passed on to us by Yang Luchan (1795–1872), we find that the theoretical framework as we understand it today was stated: "The [inner] energy is rooted in the feet, streams into the legs, and is guided via the hips all the way to the fingers. Feet, legs, and hips must be seen—and moved—as one unified whole. Moving in such a way allows a person—at the proper time and in the proper posture—to go on the offensive or to evade an attack. If the desire is to make an upward move, one must come from below, like somebody who wants to pull out a small tree: First he pushes down to loosen the roots, and then it is easy to pull the small tree out of the ground."

Two Mirror-Image Movement Combinations from Form 4

Movement combinations are a series of rhythmically flowing acyclical movements that have been strung together, as shown in the photos on pages 48 and 49.

The position shown in photo 7 (the end phase—moving to the left) suggests that the body weight has already been shifted and the muscles have been tightened for the upcoming movement (to the right) by bending the right knee. This dynamic lowering of the body through the knee bend (pushing the leg "into" the ground—the opposite direction of what follows in the main phase) is identical to an active backswing movement. Indeed, the position of the end phase of the previous acyclical movement (the movement preceding the one in the photos) blends into the backswing phase of the next movement.

Modern Movement Theory & Traditional Chinese Thought

In the following discussion, we want to reinforce the notion that our modern theory of movement is quite compatible with traditional Chinese thought.

A contemporary writer on the subject, M. Porkert, discussed hunting from the Chinese perspective. Hunting, he said, always includes active and passive aspects, distinguishing between a yang phase and a yin phase. The yang phase of the hunt begins

Yim & Yang Phases in Hunting

Phase	Main Function	Example: Hunting
Preparation Phase Yang in Yin	Creating an ideal situation to carry out the main phase (intention)	1. Finding the prey 2. Inserting the arrow 3. Drawing the bow
Main Phase Powerful Yang	Carrying out intention	1. Letting go of arrow 2. Arrow hits target
End Phase 1. Yin in Yang 2. Powerful Yin	Creating a passive situation or a dynamic transitional stage	1. Arrow penetrates animal 2. Animal is dead

with tracking down the animal and reaches its peak when the arrow is released. If the arrow hits its target and pierces the prey, the active phase changes to the passive phase (yin phase). The passive phase continues as the injury causes the animal to bleed to death. This phase gives rise to new possibilities and new activities (of a yang nature).

Porkert, however, delineated further subtleties in the yin and yang phases of the hunt. Preparing the weapon for the shot (drawing the bow and inserting the arrow) is considered yang in yin, while from the moment the arrow leaves the bow until it reaches the target is a time of powerful yang. When the arrow penetrates the animal, where active energy is absorbed, the yin phase begins, and the dying or dead animal can be seen as representing powerful yin.

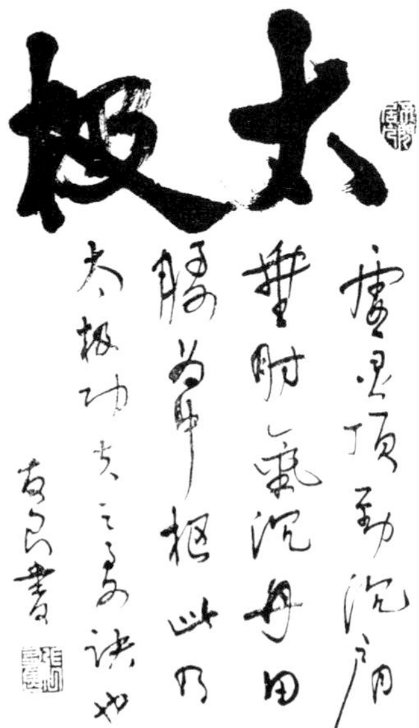

Letting go of all thought,
dropping shoulders and arms,
breathing deeply from the belly,
moving from the hips:
these are the principles of
Tai Chi Ch'uan.
—Zhang Youliang, 1992

4
Learning Tai Chi Ch'uan & Qigong

Preconditions for Learning & Training

• Tai Chi Ch'uan and Qigong can be performed regardless of age, constitution, or condition.
• People with asthmatic problems should, just to be on the safe side, consult with their physician before starting Qigong. There are no restrictions for healthy people.
• Space requirements are minimal. For Qigong, about 3 square feet (1 square meter) is all that is needed; for Tai Chi Ch'uan, a 12 × 4¼ foot (4 × 1.5 meter) space is sufficient. If you want to do Tai Chi Ch'uan at home and you have limited space, it is very acceptable not to do all the sequences; choosing individual forms is perfectly okay. However, if at all possible, try to do both exercises outside.
• To learn the exercises, it's best to spend 20 to 30 minutes practising them twice a day—right after getting up in the morning and one hour before retiring for the night. Of course, adjustments can be made to fit personal needs and schedules.
• Because of the simplicity of the Qigong exercises and the relatively small space they require, Qigong can be practised independently of Tai Chi Ch'uan; however, both are ideal for providing the body with oxygen quickly and effectively.
• Clothing requirements are also very simple: basically, loose clothes for unrestricted movements and light, soft sneakers.
• The four most important prerequisites for undertaking this practice are (1) *motivation*, through understanding the principles (theory); (2) a competent teacher; (3) practising in a positive group environment and pleasant surroundings; and (4) *persistence*. Just being interested is not enough.

Theoretical & Practical Preparations

1. Read the theoretical part of the book before starting the exercises—particularly the part on "Warm-Up & Preparation with Qigong" that follows. Theoretical knowledge is absolutely necessary for success.
2. Consider the Qigong exercises as part of the warm-up for Tai Chi Ch'uan. Pay special attention

to the instructions on "posture and movement," "breathing technique," and "guiding Chi." Then, start with Exercise 1. Only after you have mastered this exercise and can perform it without difficulty should you go on to the next one. The Qigong portion should be done, when it is part of the overall exercise program, for about 10 minutes.

3. When starting the Tai Chi Ch'uan exercises, first study the hand forms, the criteria for posture, and the positions/steps for the feet/legs.

4. Then do the preparatory exercises in the following order:

• Practise the steps.

• Do the "footwork" as part of the whole form.

5. Do a few light stretching and relaxation exercises before beginning the Qigong exercises.

Warm-Up & Preparation with Qigong

Basic Components of Qigong

These exercises originated in the area around Shanghai. They were selected by Lin Boyan, who, at this writing, is the director of the Department of Sports History at what is now the Beijing University of Physical Education (formerly the Institute of Physical Education); he is also pictured in the photos on pages 59, 61, and 63 demonstrating the exercises.

In the context of Tai Chi Ch'uan, these exercises serve as a warm-up as well as set the stage for relaxation; they also serve as a basis for learning the proper breathing techniques. The beginner should first become familiar—in theory—with the following components of Qigong:

• Posture and movement
• Breathing technique
• Concentration and guiding the Chi

Posture and Movement

Qigong exercise can roughly be divided into two categories: *exercises without moving* and *exercises in motion.* Depending on the goal, they can be practised either lying down, sitting, standing, or walking. The method we are considering here belongs to the second category, exercises in motion, and they are carried out while *standing.* The goal of this method is to learn the proper breathing technique (the proper breathing cadence) as well as to "train the Chi."

Proper breathing supports and

guides the movements (to which it is correlated), and it promotes oxygen intake and the exchange of gases within the pulmonary alveoli.

Breathing Technique

In the context of this book, we won't go into a detailed description of the anatomical and physiological process of breathing, but we still would like to point out to the beginner the essential aspects of what is meant by breathing properly to support good health, and which we highly recommend learning and using when performing Qigong exercises.

The basis of this process is the true "natural" breathing that has also been recognized by medical experts in the West as the optimal form of breathing. How does it work?

The essential job of breathing is carried out by the diaphragm. When the lungs fill up with oxygen during *inhalation*, the muscles of the diaphragm contract and the "roof" of the diaphragm is lowered, while, simultaneously, the lumbar region and the belly expand. During *exhalation*, the muscles of the diaphragm relax, returning it to its domed shape; the muscles of the belly also contract. At the end of exhalation, the abdominal wall takes on a slightly concave shape.

Among all the bodily functions, breathing is of singular importance because it is an autonomic function that can also be influenced consciously. We can observe our breath, as well as slow it down, speed it up, and deliberately suspend it.

The Chinese have been aware of the importance of proper breathing for more than 2,500 years, and it is used throughout the many different forms of Qigong exercises.

The Three-Phase Rhythm

The breathing rhythm for our Qigong exercises proceeds in three stages that are continuously repeated:

- Inhalation
- Exhalation
- Pause

1. Inhalation takes place gently but *actively* through the nose. The movements, particularly the arm movements, are synchronized with the flow of the breath. The change from exhalation to inhalation is gentle and without an attempt to control it.
2. Exhalation, again synchronized with the movements, takes place through the mouth, with the lips just slightly separated. Used-up air is *evenly* expelled

with a minimum of force; this can be compared to the stroke of a gong that becomes more faint until it finally falls silent.

3. The Pause that follows naturally is the most important. During the pause, the lungs relax, the dome-shaped diaphragm has reached its highest expansion, and the sternum and ribs are in their lowest position. The pause is the moment in which something new is about to be created; it's truly creative.

Our expectation alone of the next breath to come can be seen as healing. This "waiting" also entails an acceptance and subordination to the laws of nature.

The meaning of *waiting* can be understood as "pointing out attention to something." Therefore, let us direct our total *relaxed* attention to the impulse that concludes the pause and flows into inhalation.

Plato, in *Parmenides*, defined a pause as a "magical moment . . . in which 'one thing' changes from movement to rest and to rest to movement." He said, "Magical is this movement, because the moment between movement and rest does not belong to any time [to anybody]."

This creative pause when breathing, this magical moment, can be said to be our only reality—where there is neither past nor future, but only the eternal present.

One can also say that life begins when we inhale and ends when we exhale.

Guiding the Chi

Along with the breathing technique, directing the Chi is another component that requires concentration and imagination. During inhalation, we take oxygen in and, according to the Chinese, at the same time, Chi. With the help of our imagination, we allow this Chi to sink into the space of the belly, until it reaches an area called the *dantian*, located about three finger-widths below the navel. "Energy," by means of breathing and the guidance of the Chi into the belly area, is concentrated and stored there.

Breathing and the guidance of the Chi together lead to the optimal intake of oxygen. They also strengthen the organs in the pelvic area and, by noticeably centering the energy, stabilize the lower part of the body that will serve as the base for all movements, leaving the upper part of the body light and agile.

Yi, the power of the imagination, which also has great significance in the performance of Tai Chi Ch'uan forms, is trained through the constant repetition of Chi exercises. In addition, total mindfulness during the course of the workout in itself brings about a gentle turning away from the problems of everyday life, allowing for a comforting immersion into a state of calmness and relaxation.

A Gentle Beginning

Under no circumstances should you start Qigong exercises when angry or anxious. The body is the stage on which every emotion is deposited in the form of either visible or invisible muscle tension. Blockages and tension can't be overcome merely with good intention and the determination to relax. One must transfer pent-up emotions and tension into movements; that's when they are dissolved in relaxation—not in a state of quiet, something a tense person has trouble obtaining anyhow.

When tense or angry, begin with 10 minutes of light exercises—those that concentrate on mobilizing the shoulders, hips, knee joints, and feet and that stretch muscles and ligaments and stimulate the heart and circulatory system. During these exercises, try to concentrate on *the moment*, allowing relentless thoughts slowly and without force to dissipate or be pushed away.

When beginning these exercises for the first time, your breathing should be naturally gentle, flowing, and continuous. With regular training, your breathing will slow down and become deeper, allowing you to control its intensity and depth almost at will. However, this process should only be carried to the point where it feels comfortable—a sense you will develop over time.

Exercise 1

Exercising with the First Crow of the Rooster

Breath	Movement
Inhale	Stand with feet a shoulder's width apart, shoulders and arms relaxed, legs slightly bent.
Exhale	Raise arms sideways above your head, turning arms until your palms face each other. At the same time, transfer weight to the left leg, placing the inside of the right foot against the lower leg, just below the back of the knee.
Pause	
Inhale	Lower arms to shoulder height, palms pointing down. At the same time, place the left foot, a shoulder's width apart, parallel to the right foot; then place the left foot against the right lower leg, just below the back of the knee.
Exhale	Place left foot, a shoulder width apart, parallel to the right foot. Exhale, as you move your hands together in front of your face, as if squeezing a soft balloon. In the end position, the hands form a reversed V.
Pause	
Inhale	Move hands down as if pushing a ball under water. At navel height, turn hands so that palms are pointing towards each other—with arms and hands slightly curved. At the same time, lower your body by bending your legs. Straighten up again, and start the exercise from the beginning; repeat several times or go on to Exercise 2. At the end of the exercise, allow yourself to become very still and you can also breathe very slowly.

闻 鸡 起 舞

wén jī qǐ wǔ

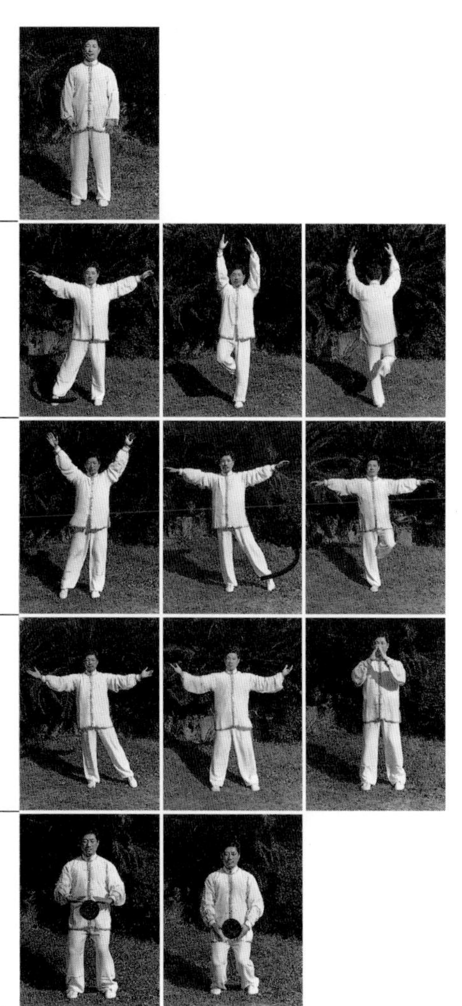

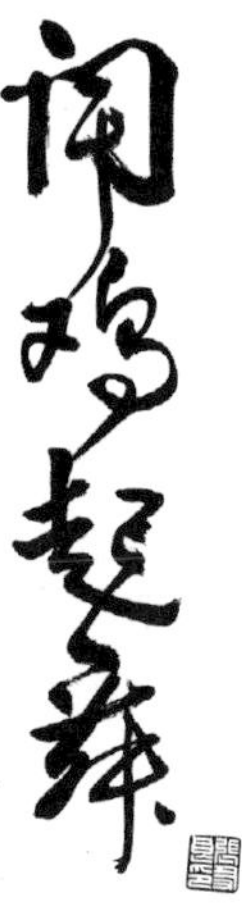

Exercise 2

Holding Up the Sun with Both Hands

Breath	Movement
Inhale	Stand with feet a shoulder's width apart, arms relaxed, legs slightly bent.
Exhale	Raise arms sideways to shoulder height.
Pause Inhale	Lower arms, slightly rounded, in front of the body with legs slightly bent. Continue moving arms and hands, slightly rounded, below the navel. Without breaking stride, bend elbows, pull up hands and forearms, and rotate them in front of the chest and the head with palms facing out in front of the face. At the same time, keep legs bent, turning hands as if you were pushing up a globe ("supporting the sun"). Look at your hands.
Exhale	Turn hands and arms so that the palms face back, while, at the same time, lowering the elbows. Palms are moved past the ears to the chest, with fingertips pointing towards each other, as if you were pushing a ball under water in front of your chest.
Pause	
Inhale	Lower hands and arms further, keeping them rounded, as if you were holding a ball in front of your stomach. Straighten up, and start from the beginning; repeat several times or go on to Exercise 3. At the end of the exercise, be still and you can also breathe slowly.

双手托日

shuāng shǒu tuō rì

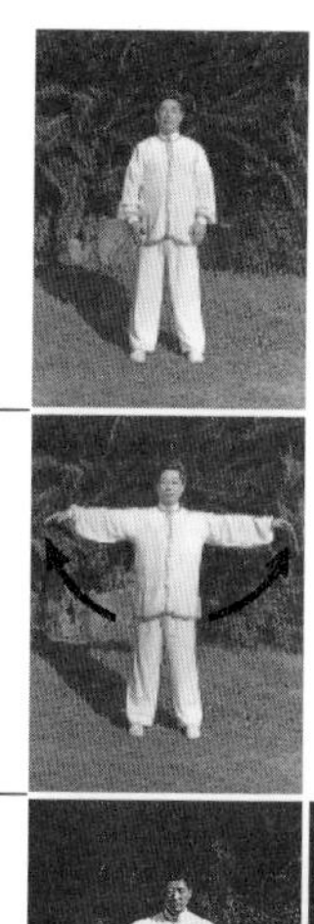

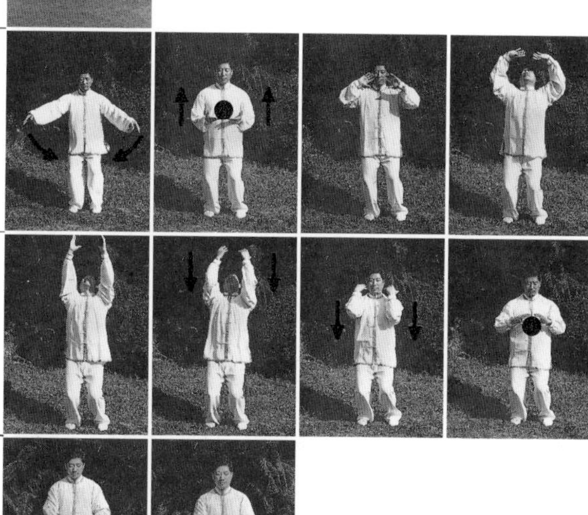

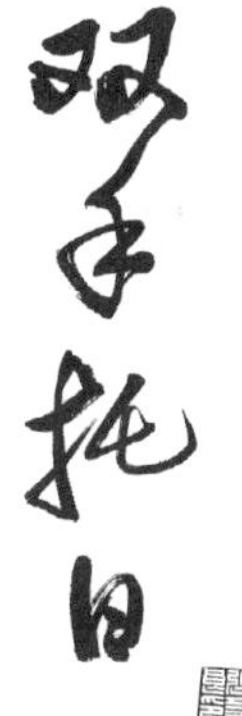

Exercise 3

Inhaling River & Mountain

Breath	Movement
Inhale	Stand with feet a shoulder width apart, arms relaxed, legs slightly bent.
Exhale	Raise arms slightly above the head, palms facing each other.
Pause	
Inhale	Move arms out to the side, slightly rounded. *Only for this exercise*, simultaneously breathe with chest and belly.
Exhale	Bend down from the waist, with legs bent. Cross hands (left hand inside for men, right inside for women); slightly raise head.
Pause	
Inhale	Move arms out at shoulder height, while slowly straightening up the upper body.
Exhale	Lift arms sideways to shoulder height.
Pause	
Inhale	Move arms sideways down in front of the body, slightly rounded, while legs are slightly bent. Cup hands below the navel; stand upright. Then start from the beginning. Repeat several times or remain in the end position, in which you can breathe slowly.

气 吞 山 河
qì tūn shān hé

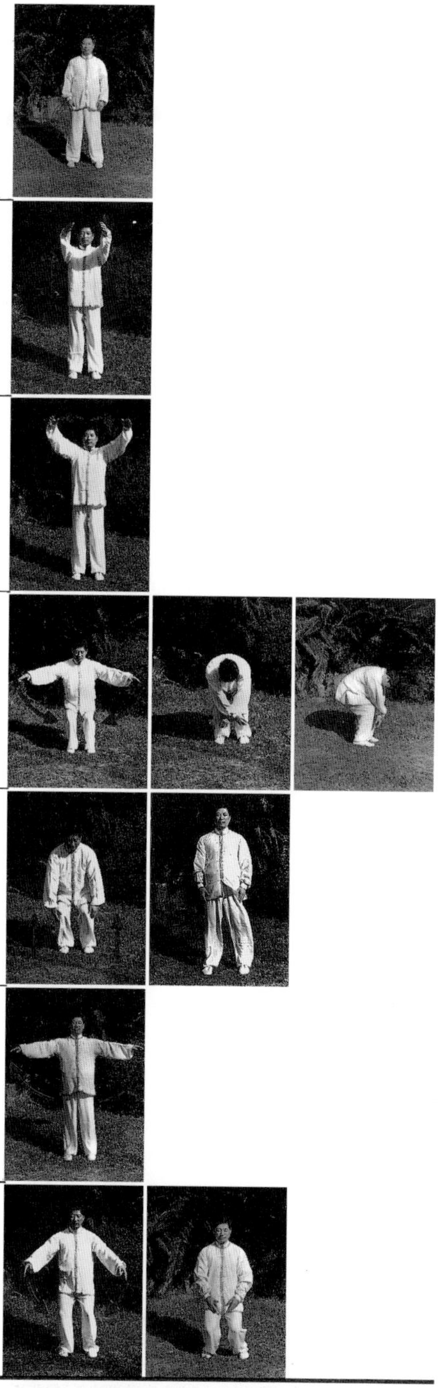

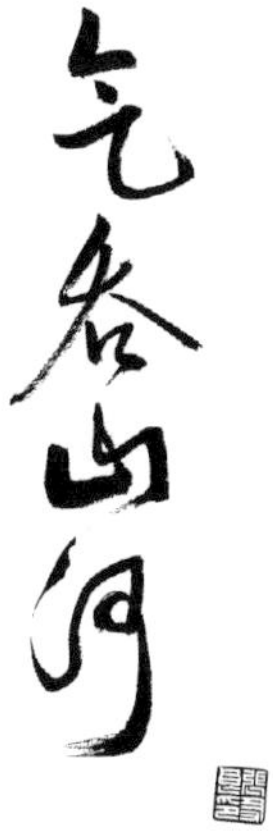

Practising Basic Tai Chi Ch'uan Movements

The Most Important Hand Movements

Since the sequences of Tai Chi Ch'uan movements are unfamiliar to beginners, it is important to take a closer look at the forms and also to practise them. Once you have learned the proper postures and movements, they should flow out from inside.

On the opposite page (65), on the left, are photos that show the movements of the hands; the photos on the right show the hand movements within the context of an exercise.

The Tai Chi Hand

Fingers are held apart and relaxed.
Wrist is relaxed.

Form 15 Left Heel Kick

The Tai Chi Fist

Hand gently makes a fist.
Fingers are not tightly squeezed together.

Form 14 Hitting Your Opponent with Both Fists

Tai Chi Dropped Hand

The thumb touches the other four fingers.
The dropped hand is relaxed and hanging down.

Form 17 Crooked Whip—Right (also called Climbing Down & Standing on Your Right Leg)

Hand Movements

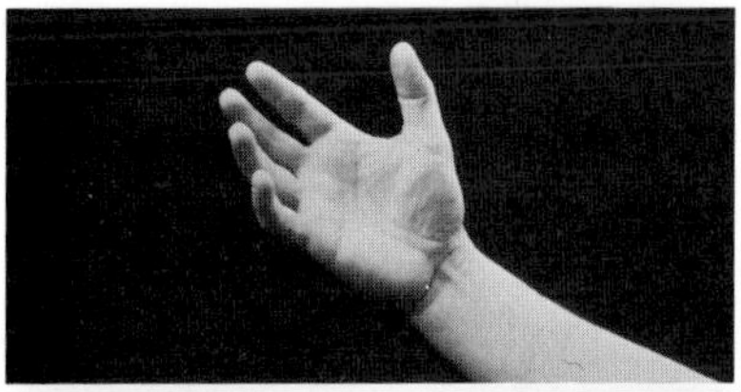

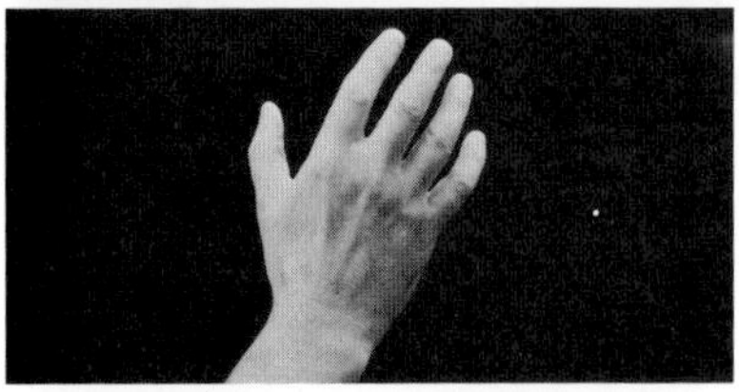

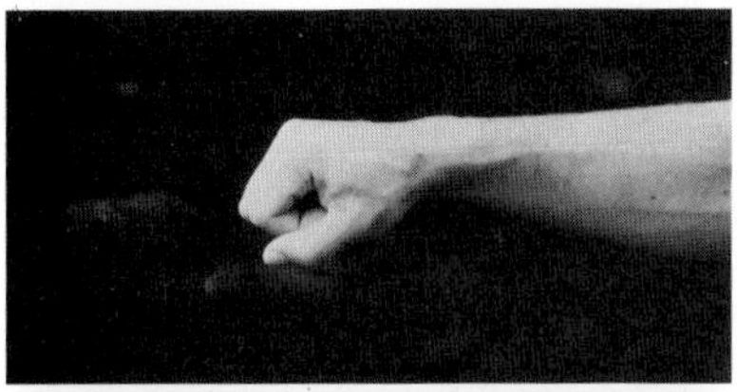

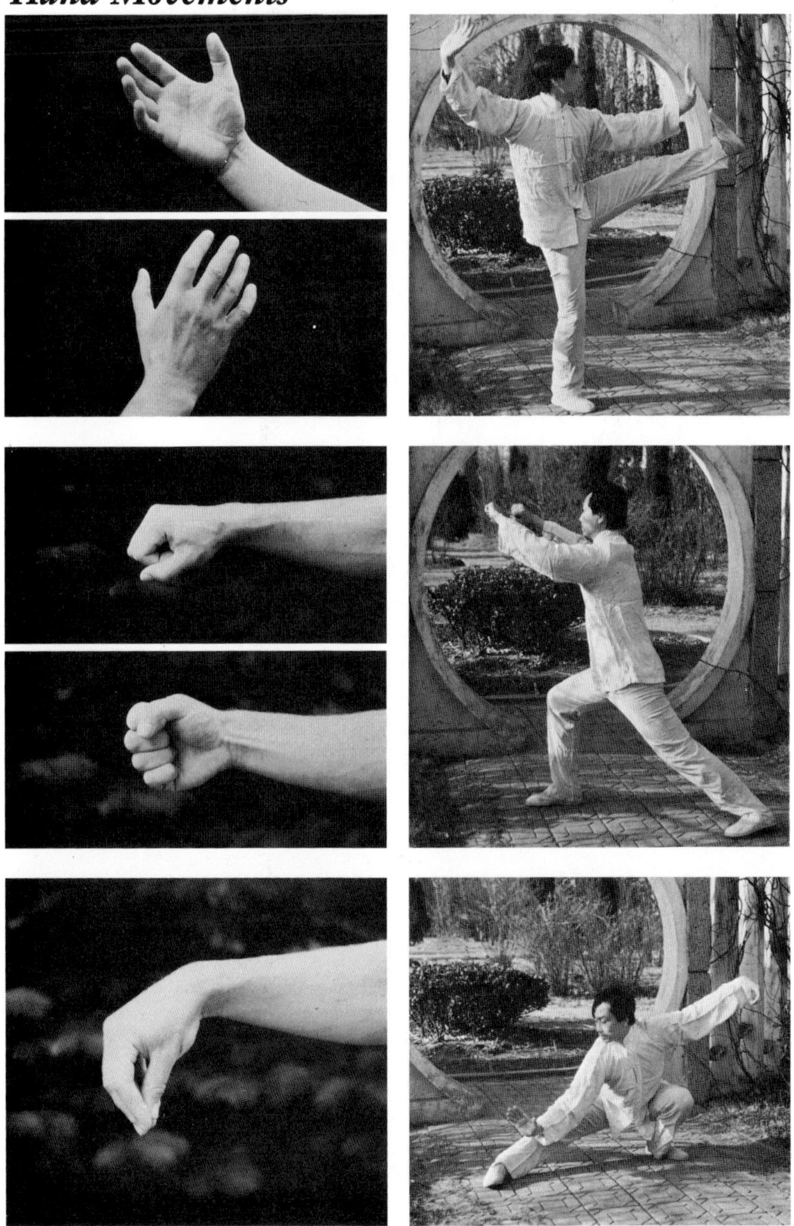

Important Criteria for Posture

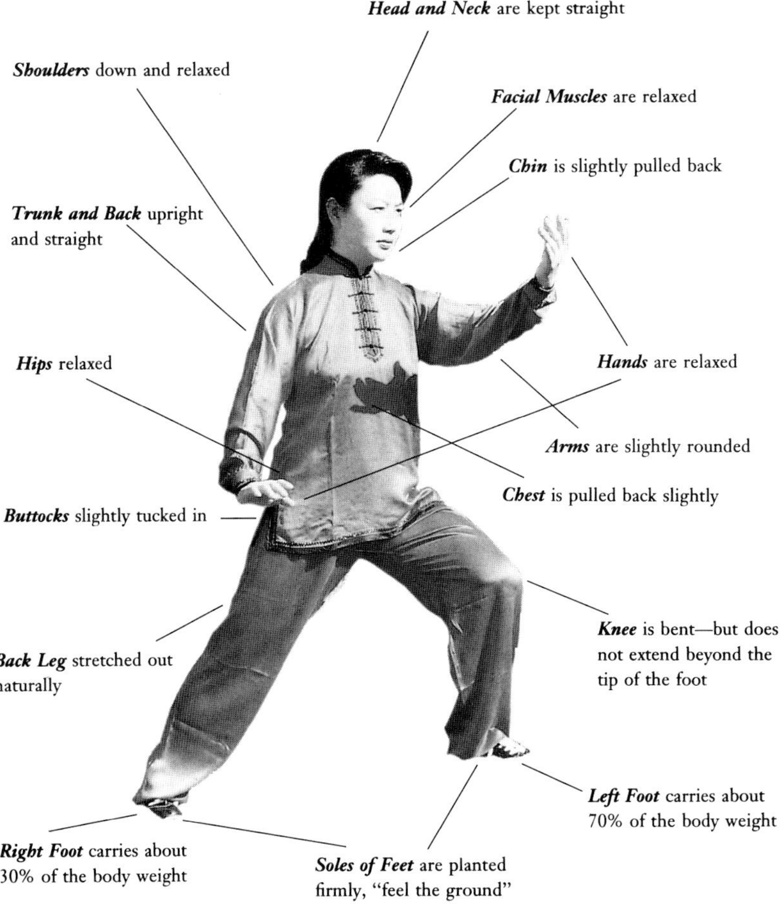
Head and Neck are kept straight
Shoulders down and relaxed
Facial Muscles are relaxed
Chin is slightly pulled back
Trunk and Back upright and straight
Hips relaxed
Hands are relaxed
Arms are slightly rounded
Chest is pulled back slightly
Buttocks slightly tucked in
Knee is bent—but does not extend beyond the tip of the foot
Back Leg stretched out naturally
Left Foot carries about 70% of the body weight
Right Foot carries about 30% of the body weight
Soles of Feet are planted firmly, "feel the ground"

Form 2 Parting the Horse's Mane

Stepping

What follows is a diagram showing types of steps, the position of the feet, the transfer of body weight, how big the steps are, and the angle of the feet to each other—all in relation to the direction in which the person is moving. We recommend that you not only study these illustrations often but that you practise the steps often too. A mirror would be an invaluable aid.

Guide to Terms & Abbreviations

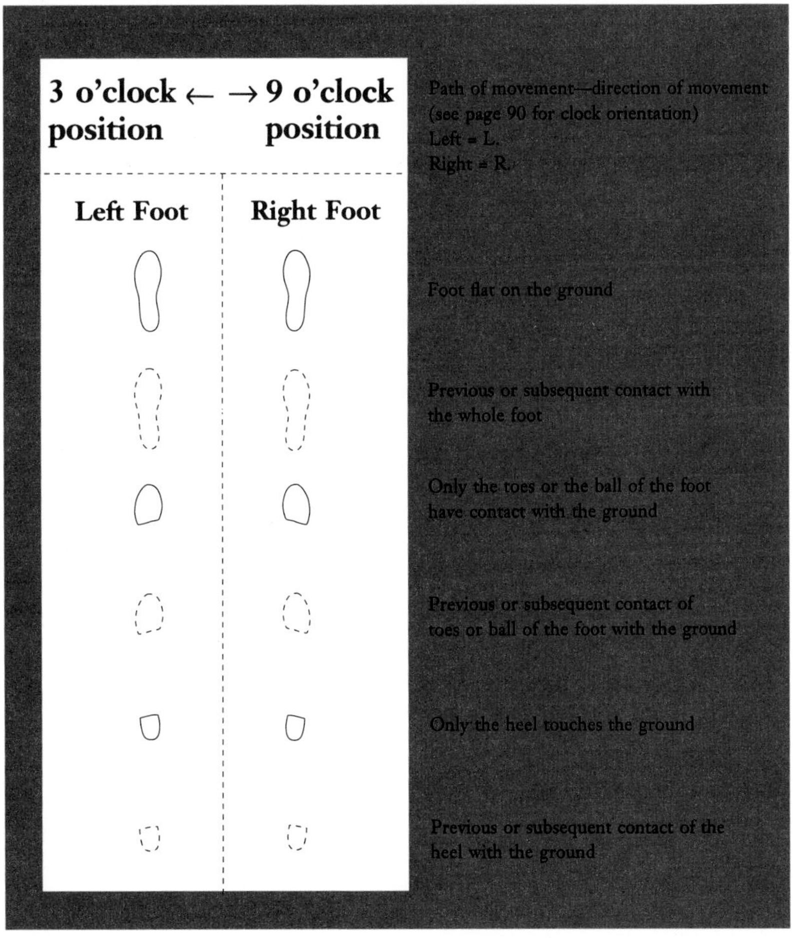

3 o'clock ← → 9 o'clock
position position

Path of movement—direction of movement (see page 90 for clock orientation)
Left = L.
Right = R.

Left Foot **Right Foot**

Foot flat on the ground

Previous or subsequent contact with the whole foot

Only the toes or the ball of the foot have contact with the ground

Previous or subsequent contact of toes or ball of the foot with the ground

Only the heel touches the ground

Previous or subsequent contact of the heel with the ground

Arched Step Forward

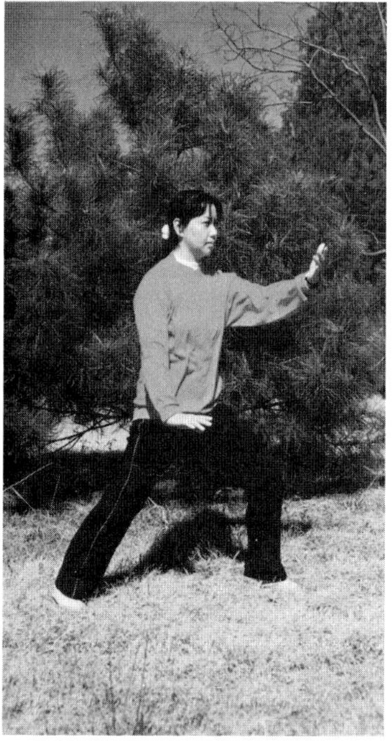

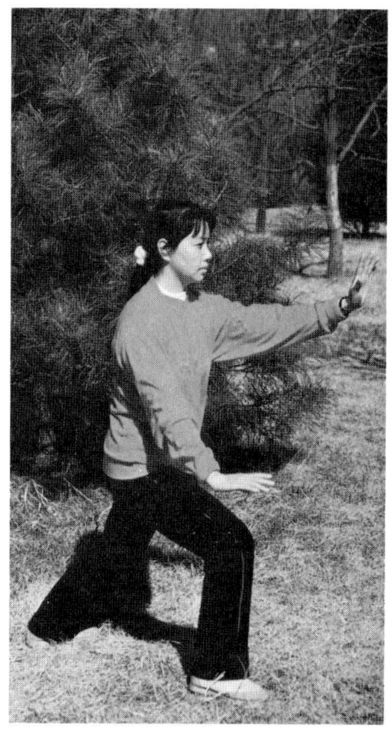

Length of step about 1¼ feet

Weight about 70%

8–12″

L. foot

R. foot

Weight about 30%

45° angle

→ 9 o'clock

Stepping to the left

Form 2 Parting the Horse's Mane

Weight about 30%

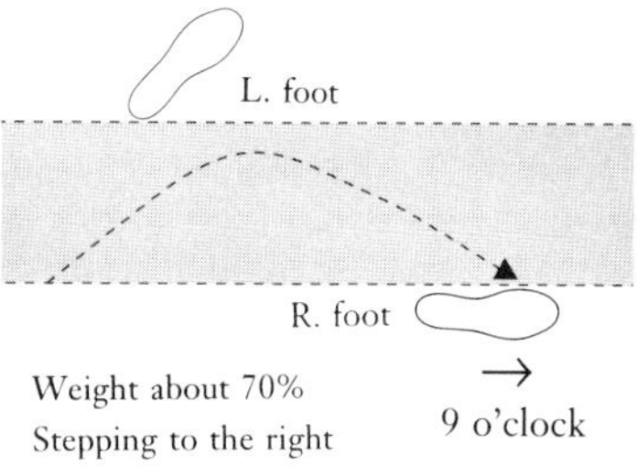

Form 4 Brushing Your Knees & Stepping

Arched Step Backwards

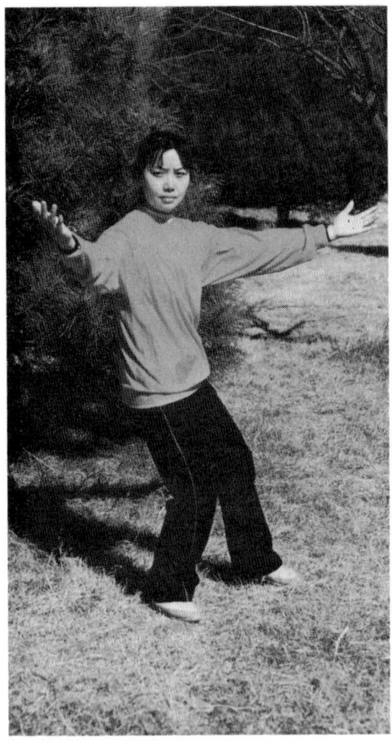

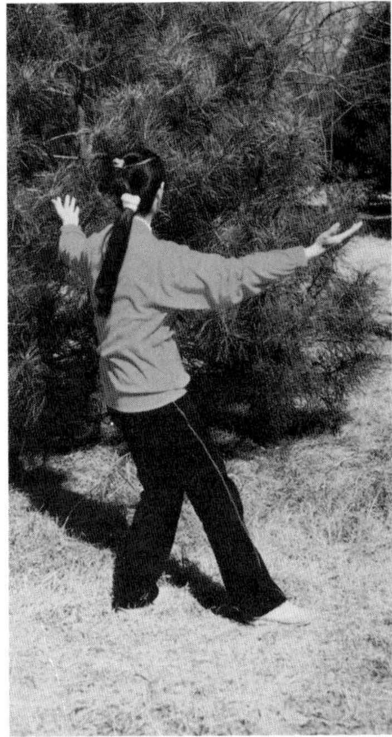

Shift weight from the L. foot to . . .

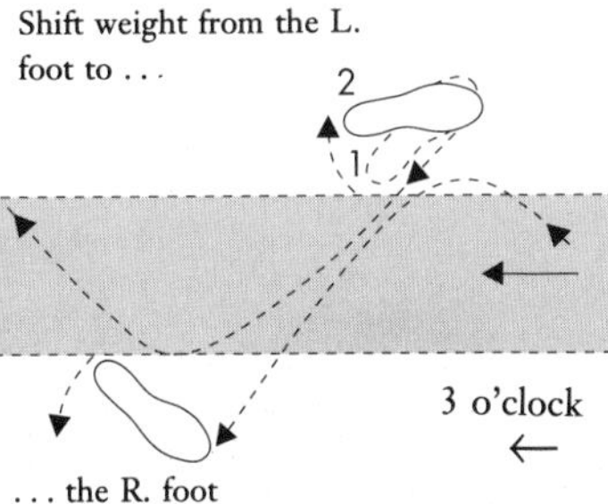

. . . the R. foot

Shift weight to L. foot from . . .

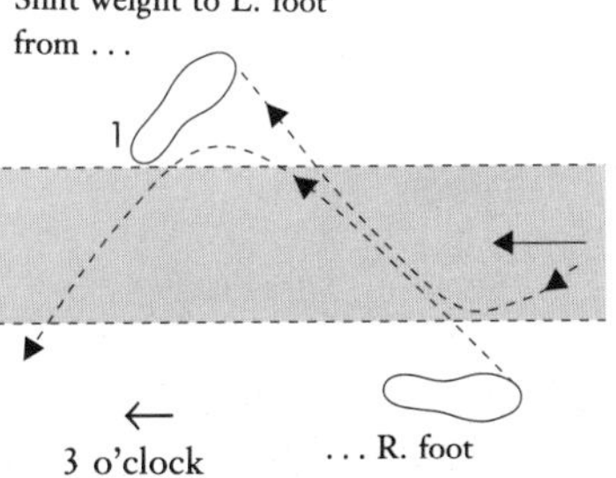

. . . R. foot

Form 6 Fending Off the Monkey

Stepping Sideways

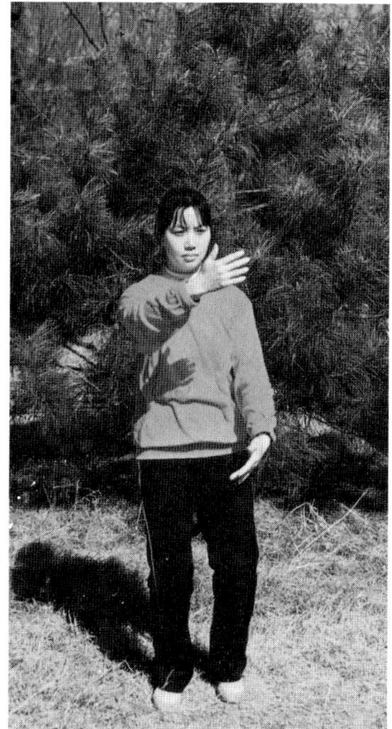

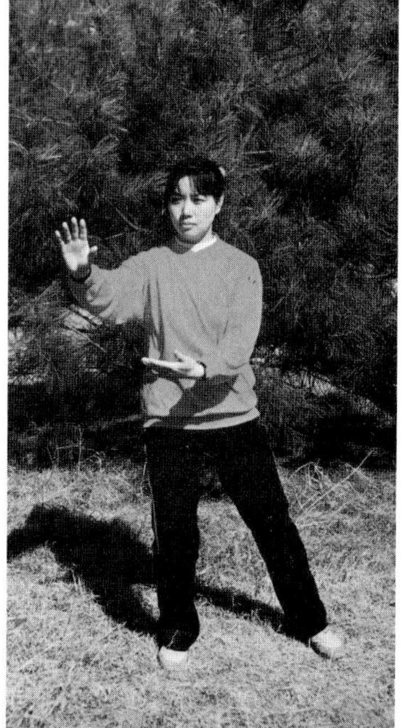

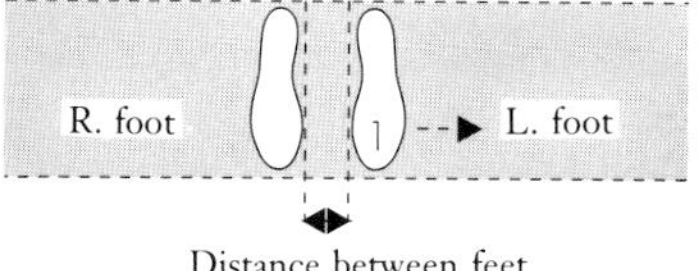

Distance between feet
width of one foot

Form 10 Moving Hands Like Clouds

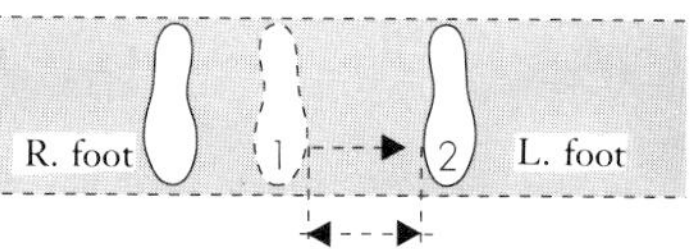

Distance between feet
width of two feet

→ 9 o'clock
Total length of step width of four feet

The Empty Step

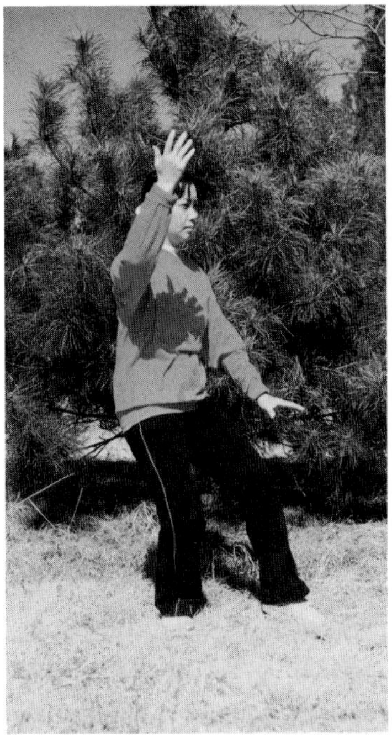

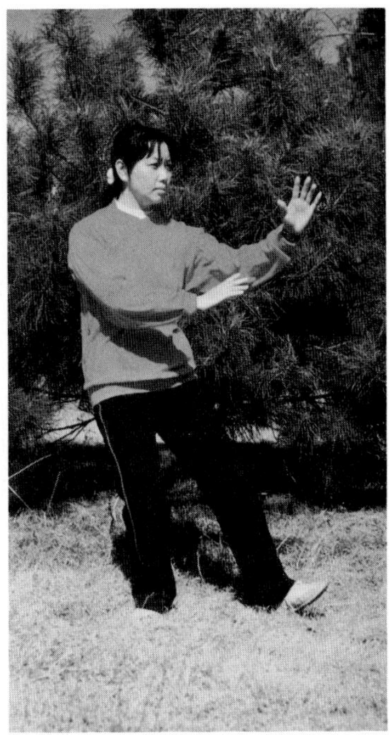

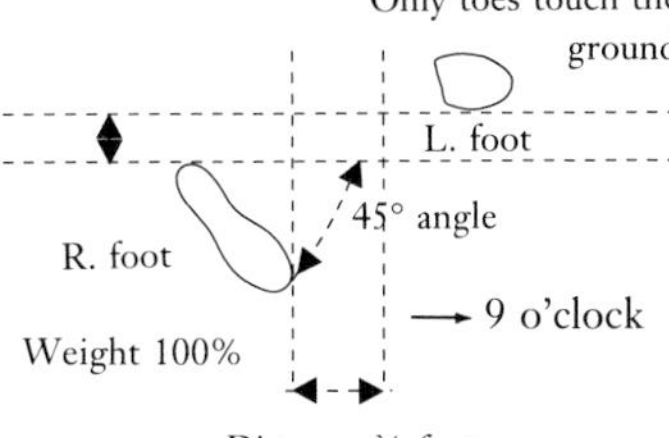

Form 3 Stork Spreading Its Wings

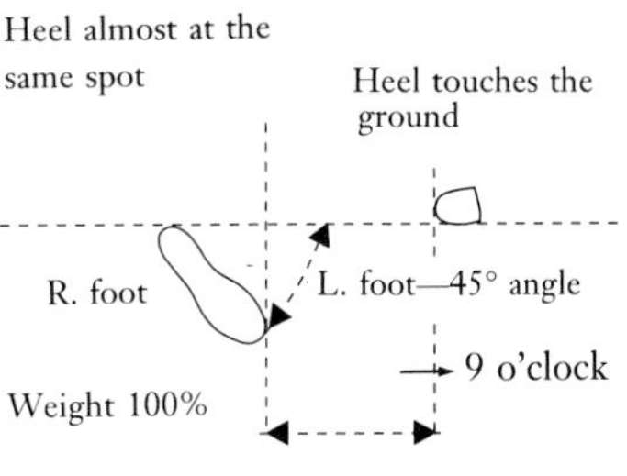

Form 5 Playing the Pipa

The Sliding Step

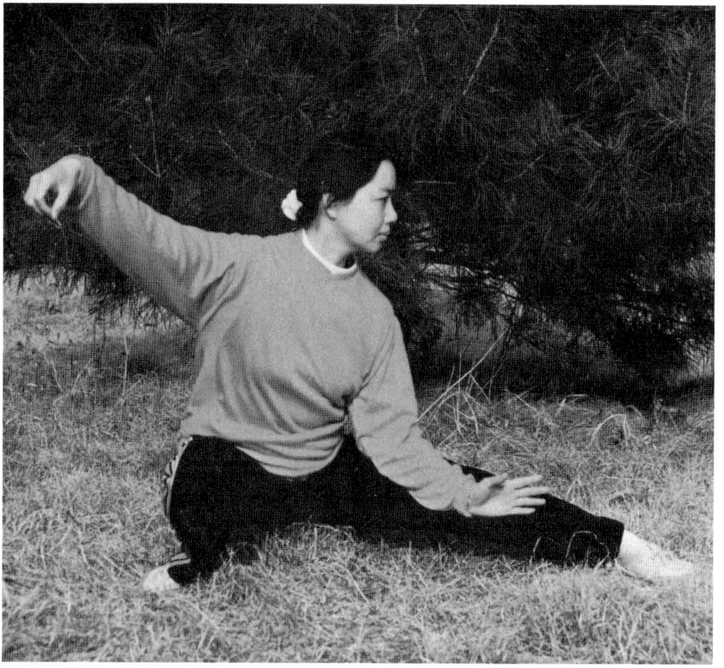

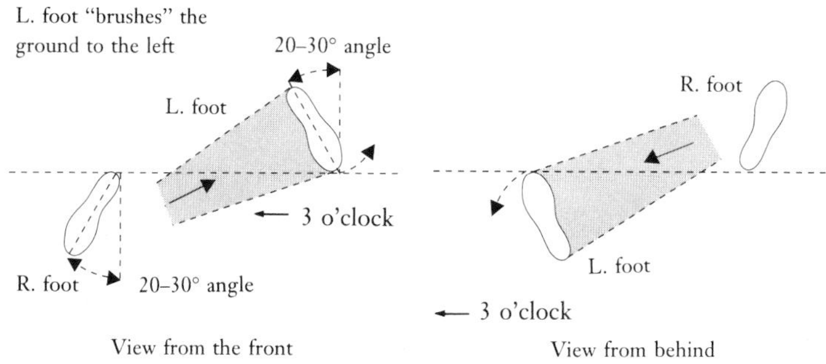

Form 16 Crooked Whip—Left

Standing on One Foot

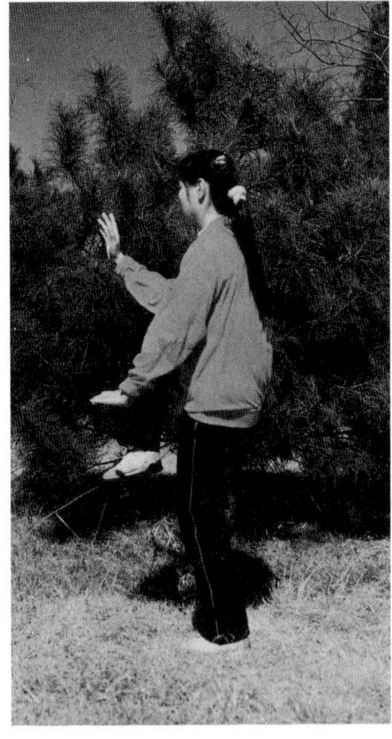

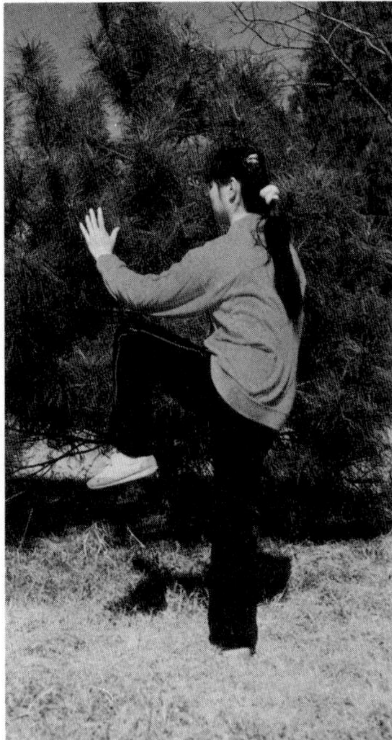

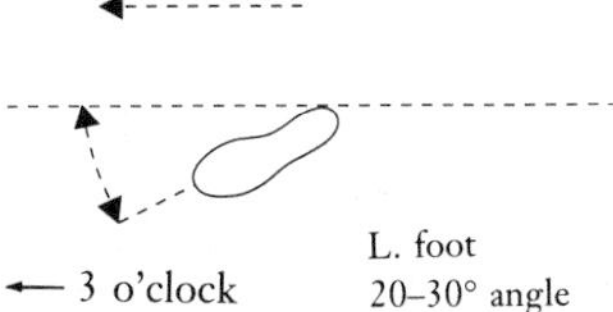

Form 16 Crooked Whip—Left

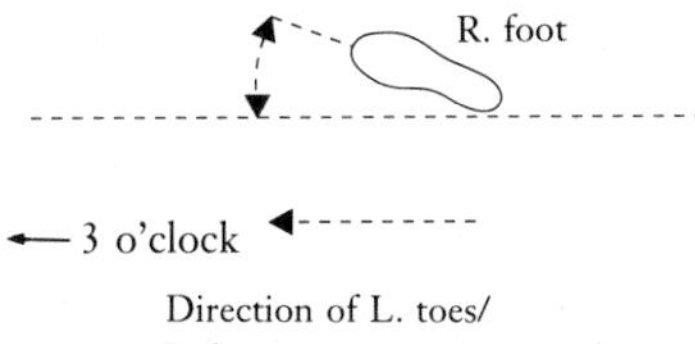

Form 17 Cracking Whip to the Right

Practising the Steps

Steps are the first actions you take when performing Tai Chi Ch'uan. The most important part is paying attention to the transfer of weight. Always make sure that the distance between the feet and the angle of the feet to each other are correct.

Exercises for Arched Step Forward

Start by relaxing your shoulders, placing your hands on your hips, and turning your eyes and your body in the direction of the movement.

a. The right foot is rotated 45° in the direction of the movement and carries the full weight. The left foot is pulled towards the right leg and touches—only in the starting position—the ground lightly. Bend the right leg before taking the first step, so that the knee and toes are approximately in line. The legs are bent—left and right—throughout the whole exercise.

b. As you turn slightly in the waist to the left, make half of an arching step to the left, placing the heel on the ground (1). Slowly lower the foot to the ground, pushing the left knee forward and transferring the weight to the left leg. Stretch the right leg as the left knee moves forward. Weight distribution: front 70 percent, back 30 percent. (See "Arched Step Forward," Form 2, page 68.)

c. Transfer the weight to the right leg, rotating the left foot on the heel about 45° to the outside (2). Move the left foot slowly to the ground, and transfer the full weight to the left leg.

d. Pull the back leg towards the right without touching the ground (3).

e. Without stopping, make half of an arched step to the right, touching the ground with the heel first; then move the knee forward in the direction of the movement, until the whole foot is flat on the ground. Stretch the back leg (see "Arched Step Forward," Form 4, page 68). Continue with c, only reverse *right* to *left* (4), with the arched step to the left (5), and so forth.

Note: Do not neglect turning the waist. Transferring weight from one leg to the other always is done with fluid motions.

Exercises for Arched Step Forward

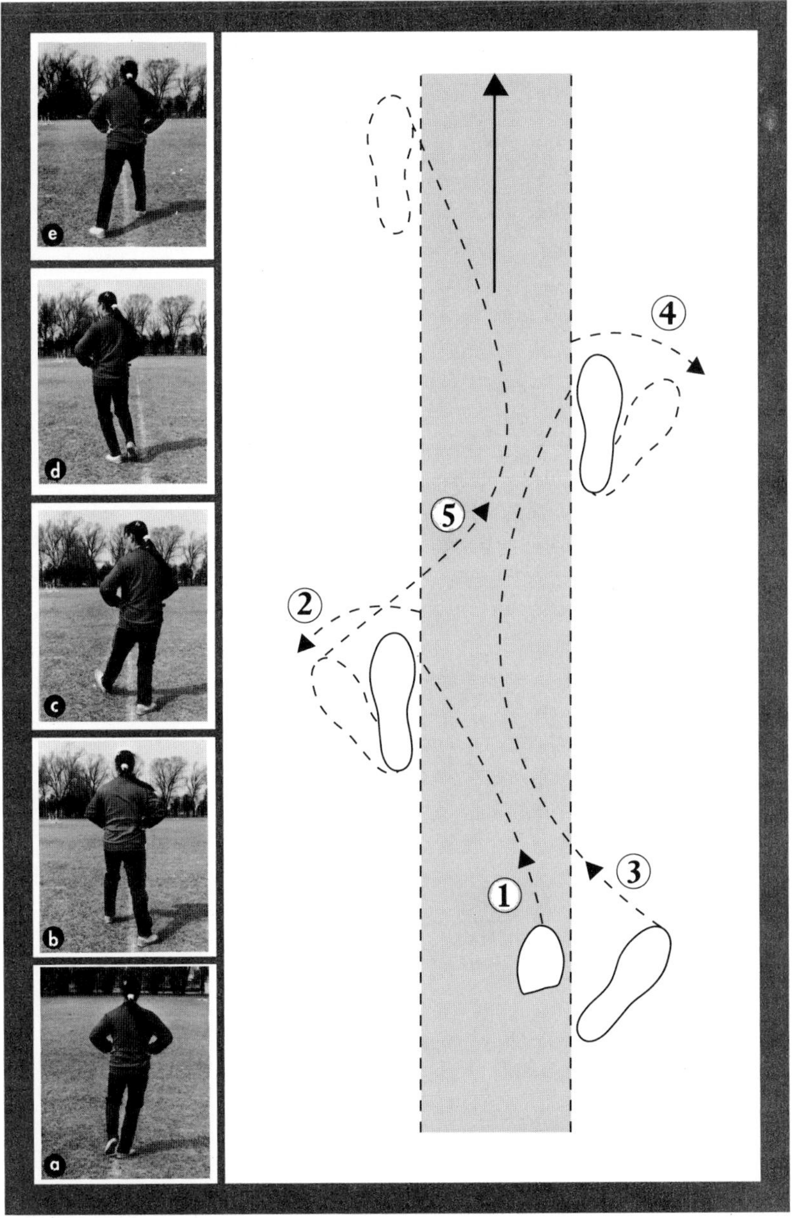

Exercises for Arched Step Backwards

Before beginning, relax your shoulders and place your hands on your hips; your back is turned in the direction of the movement.

a. The right foot is rotated 45° in the opposite direction of the movement and carries the full weight. The left foot is pulled towards the right leg and touches—only in the starting position—the ground lightly. Bend the right leg before taking the first step, so that the knee and toes are approximately in line. Both legs are bent throughout the whole exercise.

b. As you turn slightly in the waist to the left, make half of an arching step to the left (1), placing the toes on the ground first and then rolling the whole foot in a 45° angle to the ground. Transfer the weight to the left leg (see "Arched Step Backwards," Form 6, right photo, page 69).

c. With the weight shifted to the left leg, rotate the right foot on the ball of the foot to the outside (2). Move the body at the same time slightly to the right.

d. Pull the right leg towards the left without touching the ground (3).

e. Without stopping, take half of an arched step backwards, touching the ground with the toes first, and—at a 45° angle—lower the whole foot to the ground, while shifting all the weight to the right leg. The left heel rotates the foot on the ball of the foot to the outside (4). Continue with an arched step backwards to the left (5), and so forth (see "Arched Step Backwards," Form 6, left photo, page 69).

Note: While stepping back, try to avoid raising and lowering the body. The distance between the heels should be about about 8 to 12 inches (20 to 30 cm).

Exercises for Arched Step Backwards

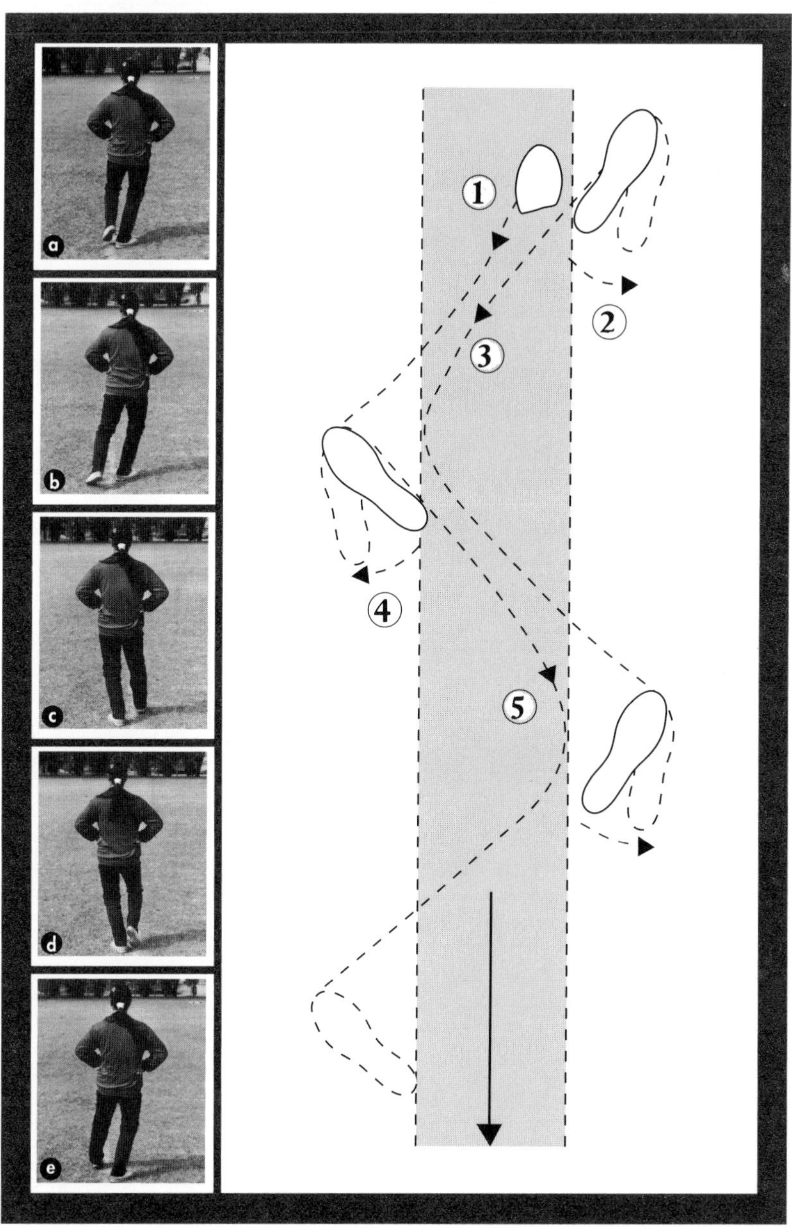

Practising Stepping Sideways

Start out by relaxing your shoulders, placing your hands on your hips, and looking straight ahead.

a. Starting position (see "Stepping Sideways," Form 10, left photo, page 70). Weight is evenly distributed on both legs.

b. Before taking the first step, bend both legs, keeping the knees and toes aligned. Step with the left leg to the left (1); the distance between the feet should be about the width of four feet. (See "Stepping Sideways," Form 10, right photo, page 70.) Gently set the toes on the ground. Then slowly roll the whole foot to the ground and transfer the full weight to this side.

c. Pull the right leg to the left (2), so that the feet, again, are the width of one foot apart.

d. Transfer the weight to the right leg, and continue to the next step.

Also practise "stepping sideways" to the right side.

Practising Stepping Sideways

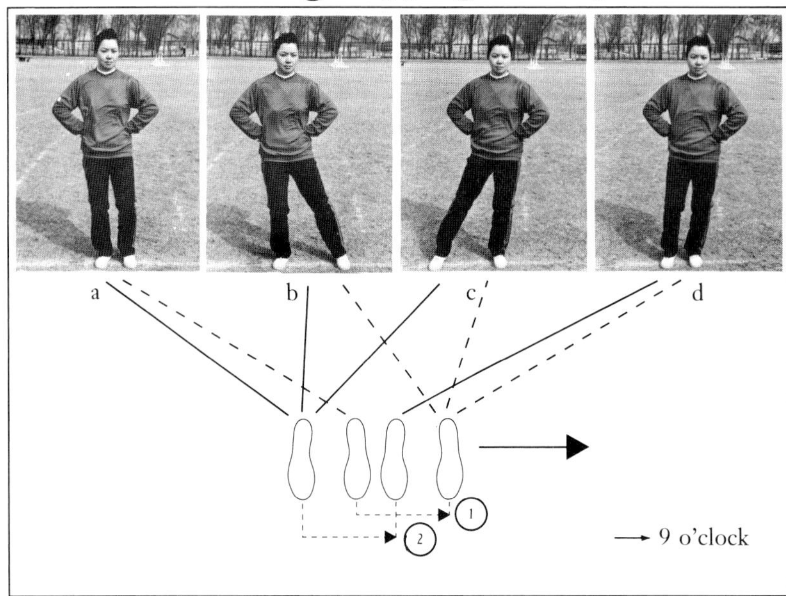

Stepping Exercises for the Entire Form

Before performing the complete sequence, practise the steps in the entire form that we have chosen here several times, on a longer path. The length of the path should be gauged by the distance of the movement. Concentrate on following the steps mindfully and exactly, paying special attention to the rotation of the body. These will help you practise Tai Chi Ch'uan gracefully.

Tai Chi Ch'uan Class

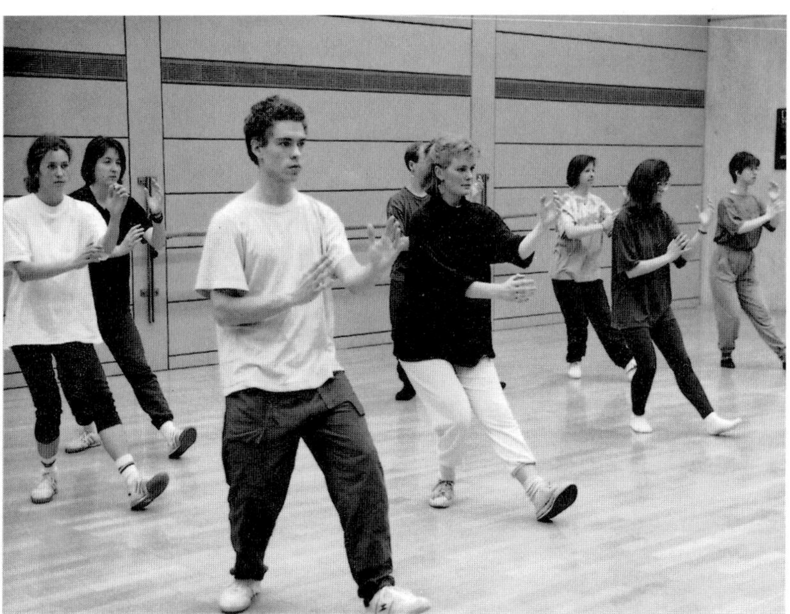

Stepping Exercises for Form 4

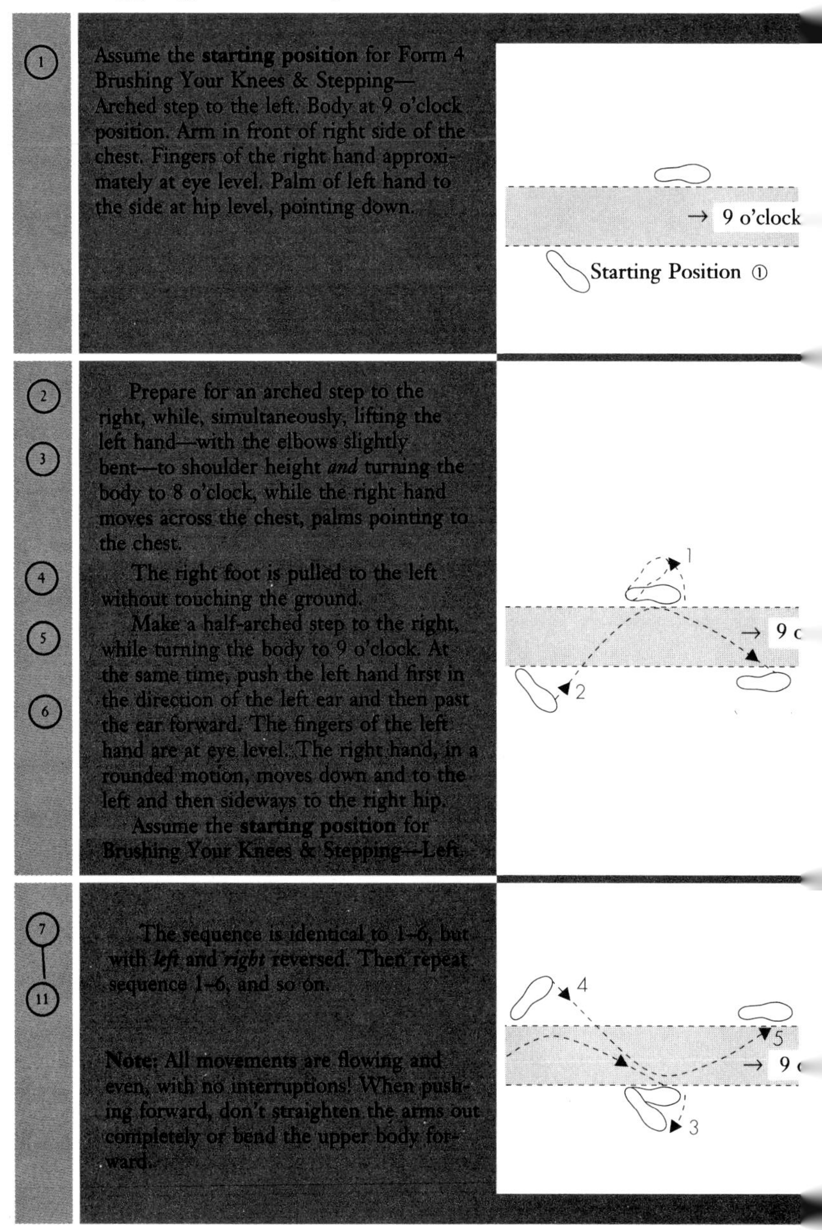

① Assume the **starting position** for Form 4 Brushing Your Knees & Stepping—Arched step to the left. Body at 9 o'clock position. Arm in front of right side of the chest. Fingers of the right hand approximately at eye level. Palm of left hand to the side at hip level, pointing down.

② ③ Prepare for an arched step to the right, while, simultaneously, lifting the left hand—with the elbows slightly bent—to shoulder height *and* turning the body to 8 o'clock, while the right hand moves across the chest, palms pointing to the chest.

④ The right foot is pulled to the left without touching the ground.

⑤ Make a half-arched step to the right, while turning the body to 9 o'clock. At the same time, push the left hand first in the direction of the left ear and then past the ear forward. The fingers of the left hand are at eye level. The right hand, in a rounded motion, moves down and to the left and then sideways to the right hip.

⑥ Assume the **starting position** for Brushing Your Knees & Stepping—Left.

⑦–⑪ The sequence is identical to 1–6, but with *left* and *right* reversed. Then repeat sequence 1–6, and so on.

Note: All movements are flowing and even, with no interruptions! When pushing forward, don't straighten the arms out completely or bend the upper body forward.

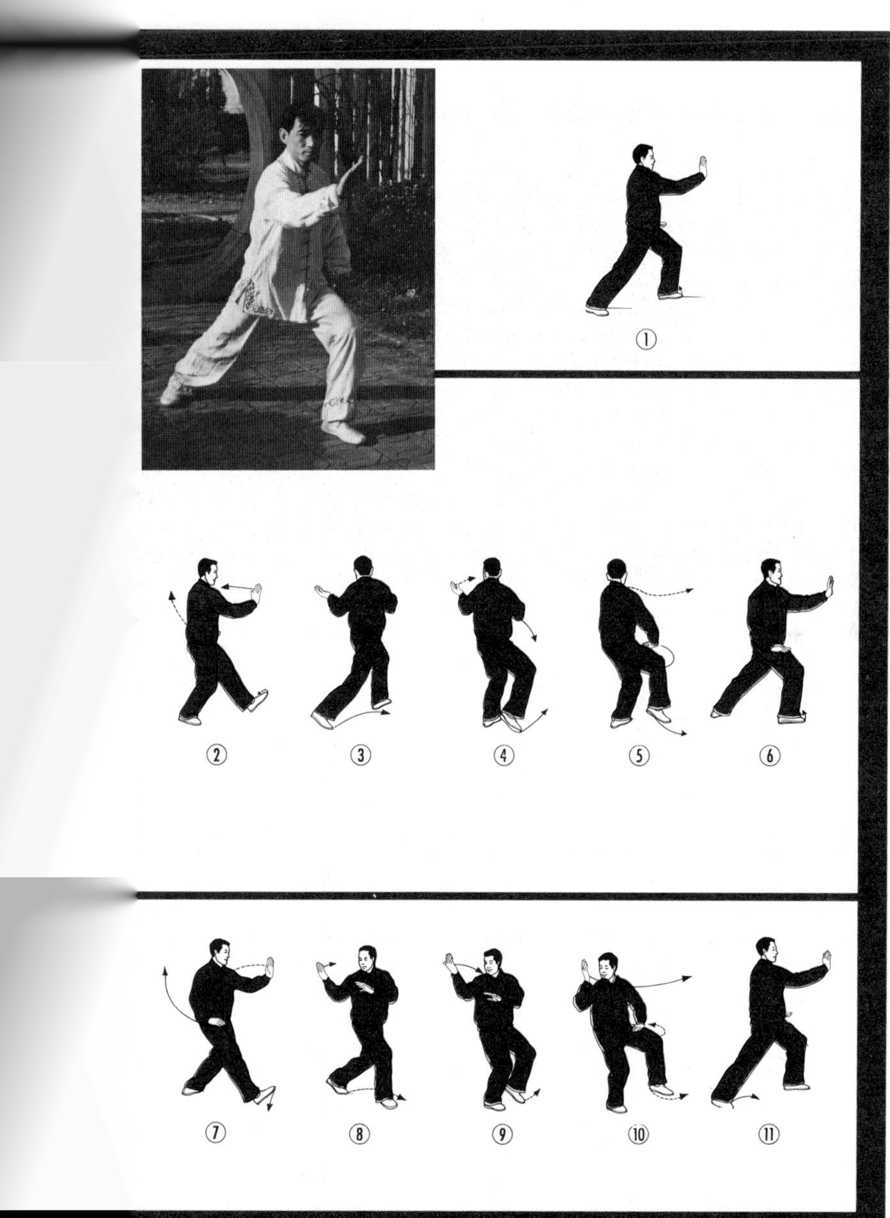
①
②
③
④
⑤
⑥
⑦
⑧
⑨
⑩
⑪

Stepping Exercises for Form 6

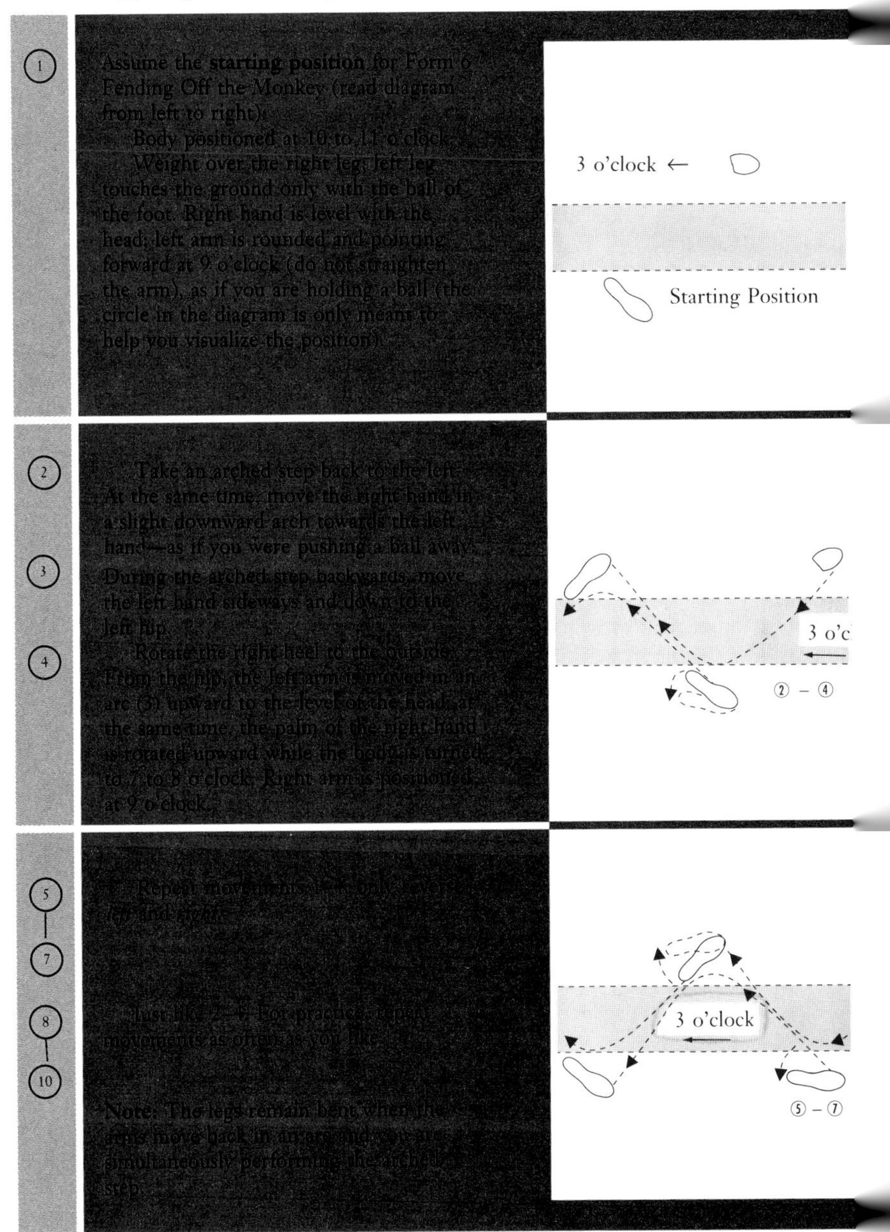

①

Assume the **starting position** for Form 6 Fending Off the Monkey (read diagram from left to right):

Body positioned at 10 to 11 o'clock.

Weight over the right leg; left leg touches the ground only with the ball of the foot. Right hand is level with the head; left arm is rounded and pointing forward at 9 o'clock (do not straighten the arm), as if you are holding a ball (the circle in the diagram is only meant to help you visualize the position).

② ③ ④

Take an arched step back to the left. At the same time, move the right hand in a slight downward arch towards the left hand—as if you were pushing a ball away. During the arched step backwards, move the left hand sideways and down to the left hip.

Rotate the right heel to the outside. From the hip, the left arm is moved in an arc (3) upward to the level of the head; at the same time, the palm of the right hand is rotated upward while the body is turned to 7 to 8 o'clock. Right arm is positioned at 9 o'clock.

⑤–⑦

Repeat movements 2–4, only reverse *left* and *right*.

⑧–⑩

Just like 2–4. For practice, repeat movements as often as you like.

Note: The legs remain bent when the arms move back in an arc and you are simultaneously performing the arched step.

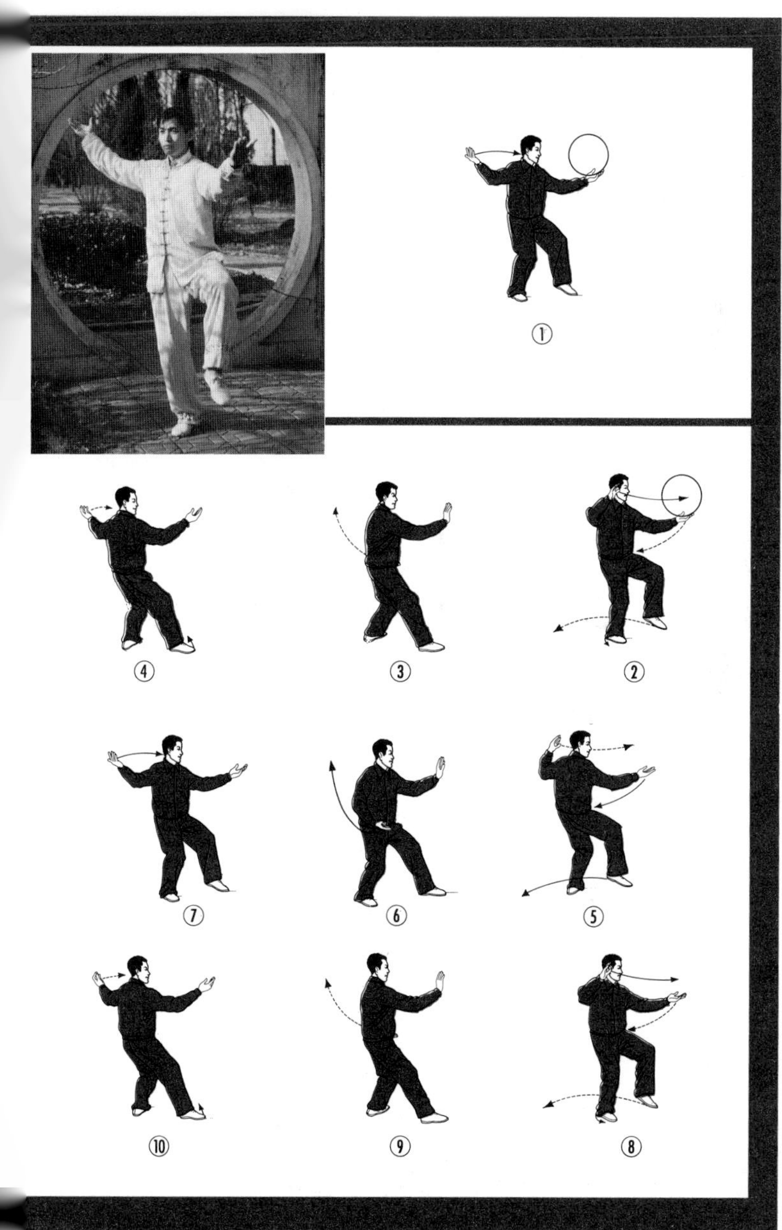
①
④
③
②
⑦
⑥
⑤
⑩
⑨
⑧

Stepping Exercises for Form 10

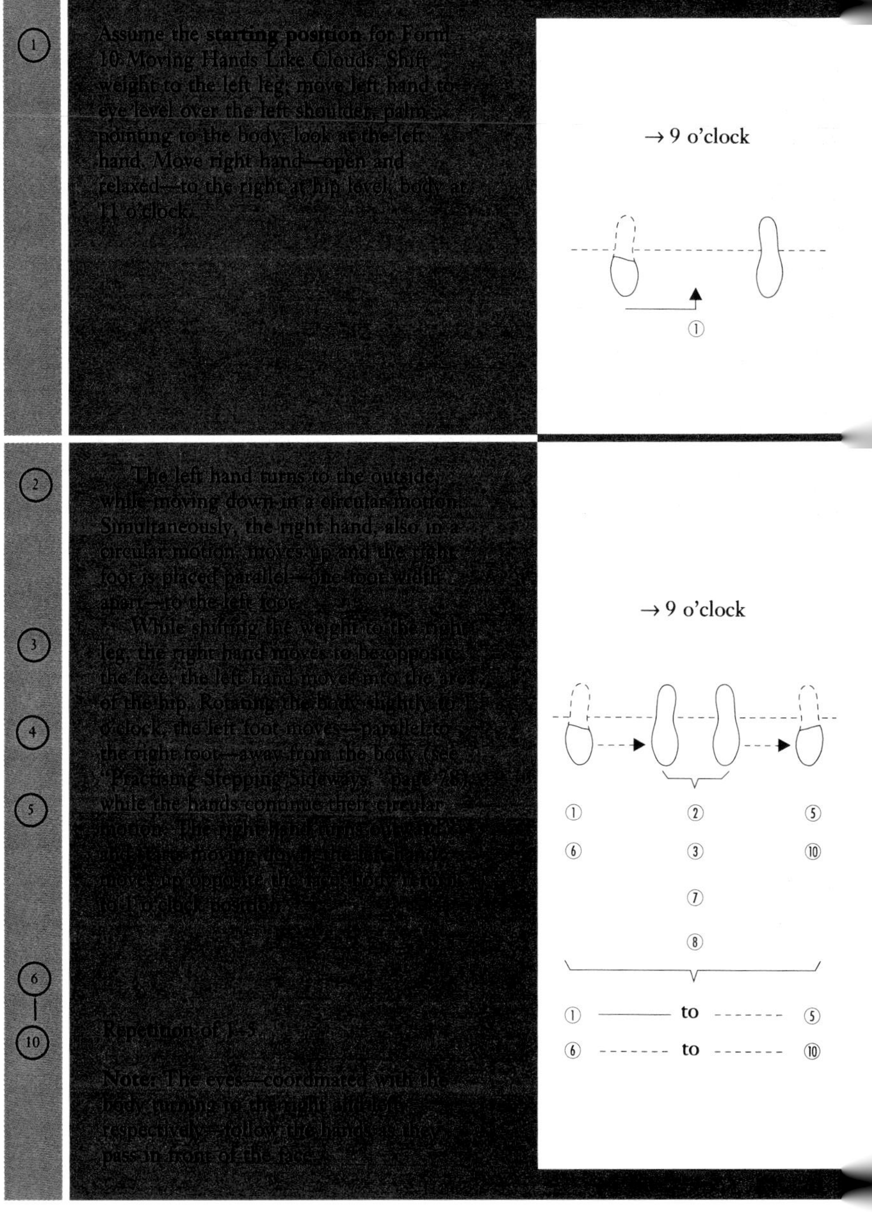

1 Assume the **starting position** for Form 10 Moving Hands Like Clouds. Shift weight to the left leg; move left hand to eye level over the left shoulder, palm pointing to the body; look at the left hand. Move right hand—open and relaxed—to the right at hip level, body at 11 o'clock.

2 The left hand turns to the outside while moving down in a circular motion. Simultaneously, the right hand, also in a circular motion, moves up and the right foot is placed parallel—one foot width apart—to the left foot.

3 While shifting the weight to the right leg, the right hand moves to be opposite the face, the left hand moves into the area of the hip. Rotating the body slightly to 1

4 o'clock, the left foot moves—parallel to the right foot—away from the body (see "Practising Stepping Sideways," page 78),

5 while the hands continue their circular motion. The right hand turns outward and starts moving down; the left hand moves up opposite the face, body [illegible] to 1 o'clock position.

6–10 Repetition of 1–5.

Note: The eyes—coordinated with the body turning to the right and left respectively—follow the hands as they pass in front of the face.

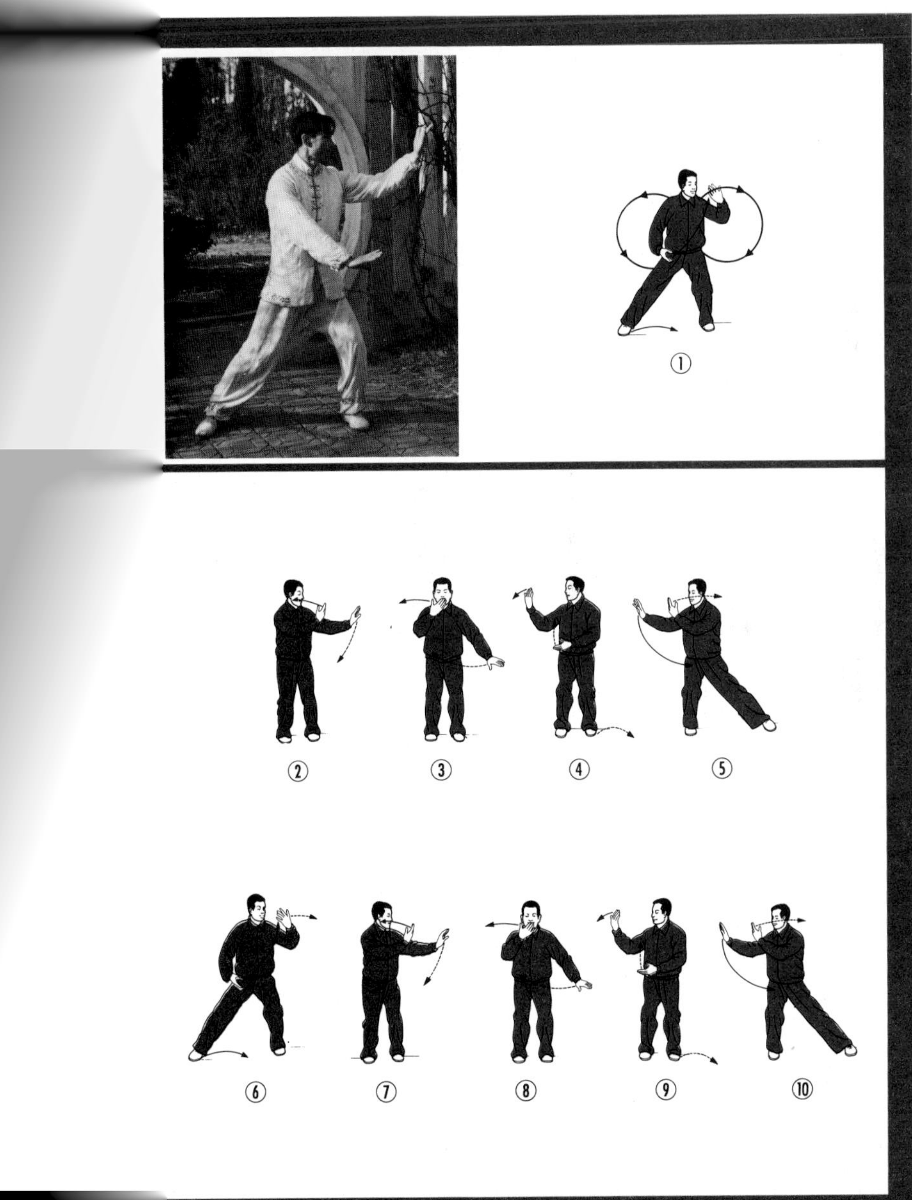
①
②
③
④
⑤
⑥
⑦
⑧
⑨
⑩

Practising Complete Sequences

Once you've studied all 24 forms and are roughly familiar with all the sequences, you can devise a one-hour exercise program as follows:

Warm-up (10 minutes)
- Jogging in place, stimulating the circulatory system
- Mobilizing joints and stretching

Qigong Warm-up (10 minutes)
Exercises 1–3

Repetitions (10 minutes)
- Practising individual and particularly difficult forms
- Practising these forms integrated with other forms

Practising the Sequences (25 minutes)
Try to do four to six sequences without stopping in between and, if possible, with deep knee bends.

Concluding with Qigong (5 minutes)
Choose any exercise.

Your goal should be, after a short warm-up, to practise the Beijing Short Form for 30 minutes with full concentration; if possible, try to practise it every day!

Many of these exercises are very simple, but it is not all that easy to become a "practitioner," which means repeating the required exercises many, many times faithfully and precisely.

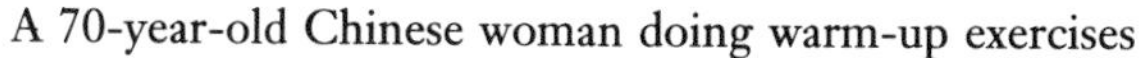

A 70-year-old Chinese woman doing warm-up exercises

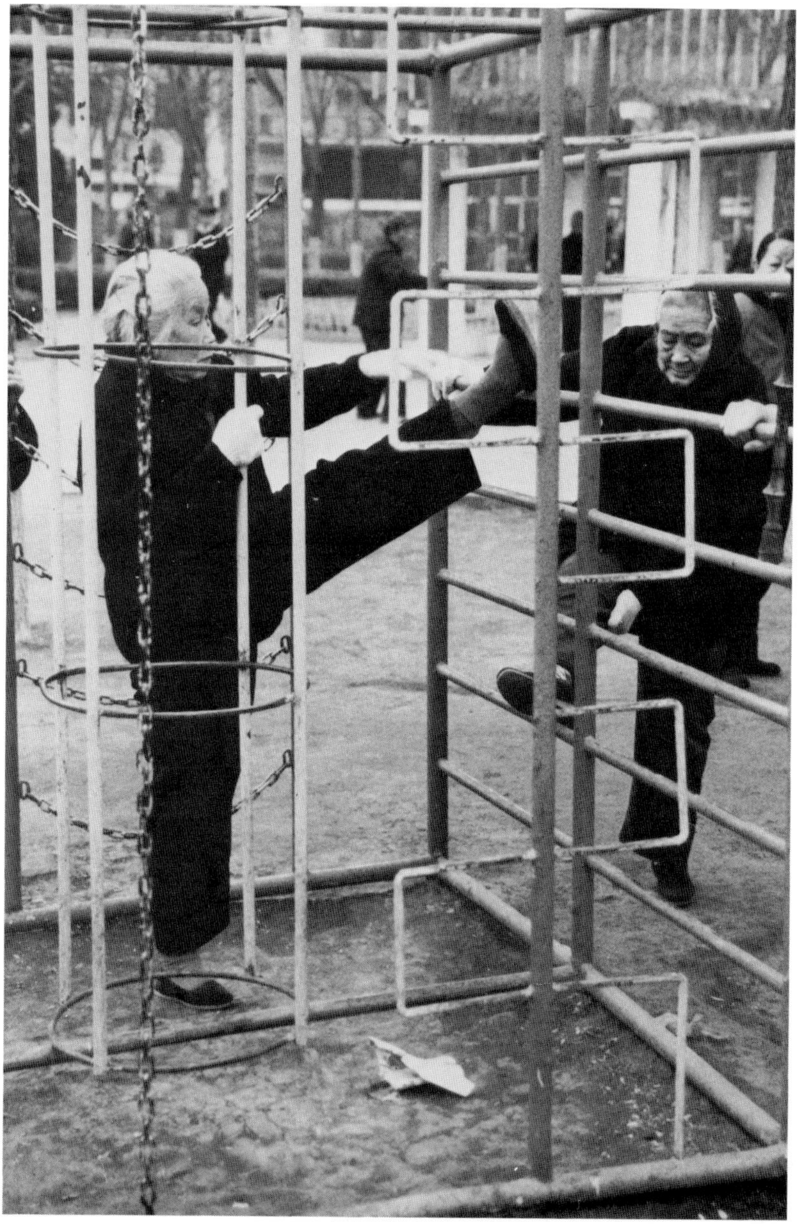

5
Beijing Short Form

Path & Forms

An Overview of the Sequences

Direction of Movement

Necessary Space
13 feet (4 m) long
4½ feet (1.5 m) wide

Path 1	**Path 2**	**Path 3**	**Path 4**	**Path 5**
9 o'clock		9 o'clock		
5 Playing the Pipa	**6** Fending Off the Monkey	**15** Left Heel Kick	**16** Crooked Whip —L.	
4 Brushing Your Knees & Stepping		**14** Hitting Your Opponent with Both Fists	**17** Crooked Whip —R.	
		13 Right Heel Kick		9 o'clock
3 Stork Spreading Its Wings	**7** Grasping the Sparrow's Tail—L.	**12** Patting the Horse's Neck While Riding	**18** Throwing the Loom—L. & R.	**24** Conclusion → 12 o'clock
		11 Simple Whip		**23** Crossing Your Hands
2 Parting the Horse's Mane		**10** Moving Hands Like Clouds	**19** Needle at the Bottom of the Ocean	**22** Closure
1 Beginning → 12 o'clock	**8** Grasping the Sparrow's Tail—R.	**9** Simple Whip	**20** Unfolding Your Arms Like a Fan	**21** Turning Around, Warding Off & Punching
	3 o'clock		3 o'clock	

Orienting the Body during Movement

The directions in which the body moves are given according to the *face of the clock.* For instance, at the beginning of a sequence the person in the photo is facing forward, with 12 o'clock behind him, 6 o'clock in front of him, 9 o'clock to his left, and 3 o'clock to his right. He has assumed an open stance from a closed stance.

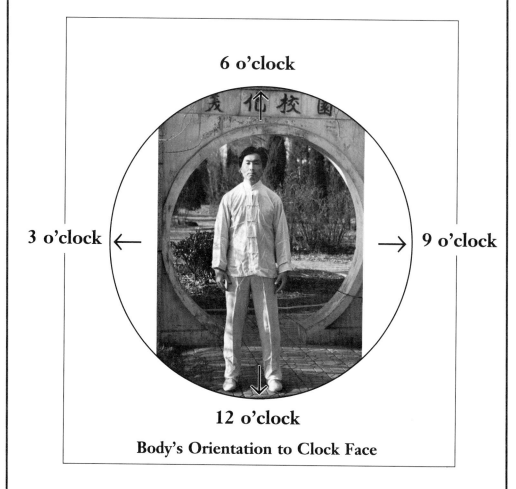

Body's Orientation to Clock Face

Descriptions of the 24 Forms

Some instructional books use as orientation the four points of the compass, where the person would be facing North. South would then be behind him, West to his left, and East to his right. But we decided to use the face of the clock, as it allows more accurate differentiation.

We recommend starting **Form 1** by always facing in the same direction. This will make the learning process and orientation easier. The pages that follow describe the 24 forms and indicate starting positions.

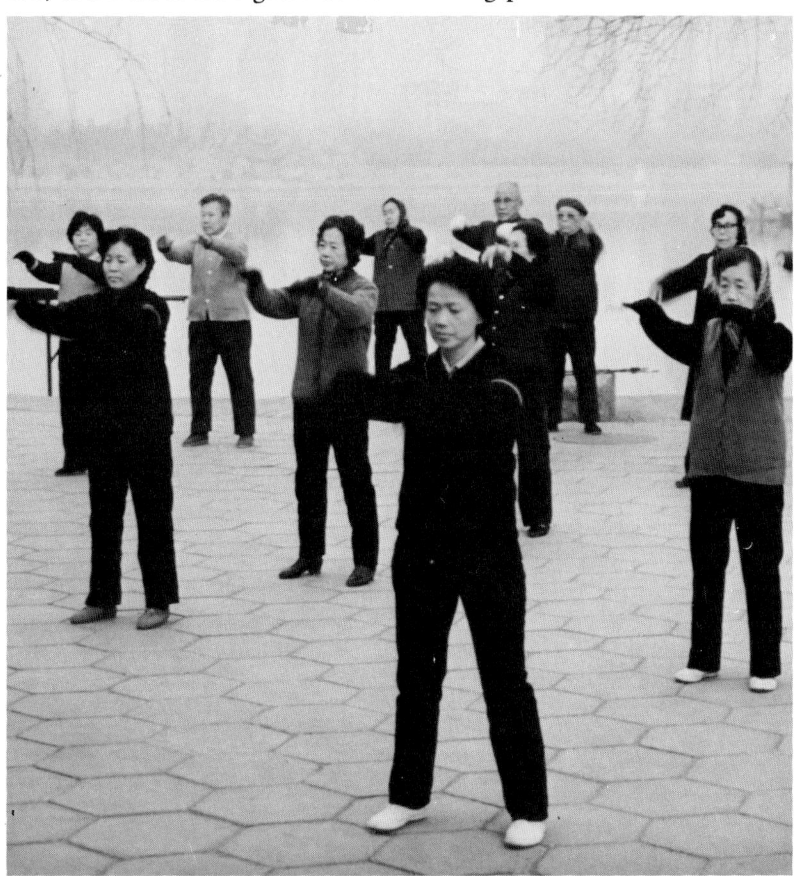

Form 1 Beginning

Beginning

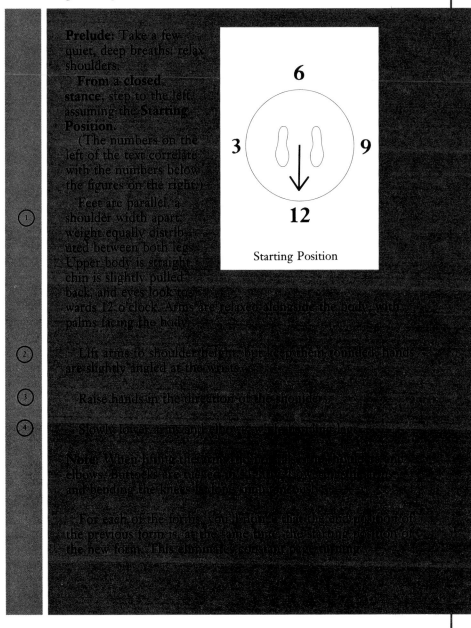

Starting Position

Prelude: Take a few quiet, deep breaths; relax shoulders.

From a closed stance, step to the left, assuming the **Starting Position.**

(The numbers on the left of the text correlate with the numbers below the figures on the right.)

1 Feet are parallel, a shoulder width apart, weight equally distributed between both legs. Upper body is straight, chin is slightly pulled back, and eyes look towards 12 o'clock. Arms are relaxed alongside the body, with palms facing the body.

2 Lift arms to shoulder height, but keep them rounded; hands are slightly angled at the wrists.

3 Raise hands in the direction of the shoulders.

4 Slowly lower arms and elbows while bending legs.

Note: When lifting the arms do not raise the shoulders [illegible] elbows. Buttocks are tucked in [illegible] and bending the knees is done [illegible].

For each of the forms, you'll notice that the end position of the previous form is, at the same time, the starting position of the new form. This eliminates constant page turning.

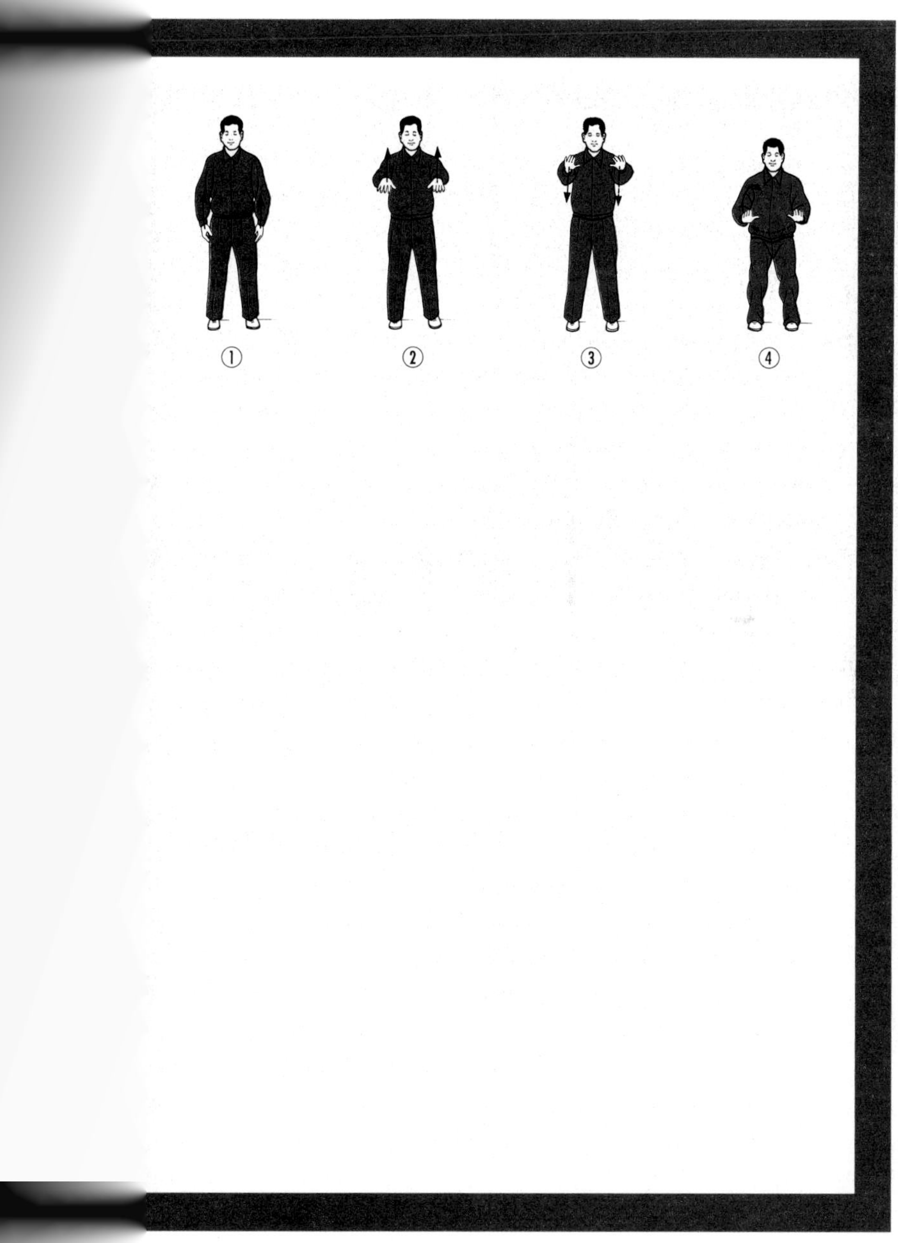
①
②
③
④

Parting the Horse's Mane

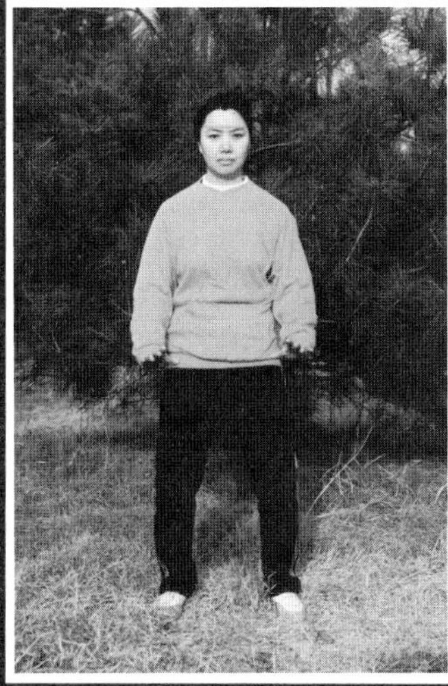

Starting Position—12 o'clock

(5) Shift weight to the left
foot, while slightly turning the upper body to
1 o'clock. At the same
time, move the right
hand up in an arc to
chest level, while mov-
(6) ing the left hand down
to the middle of the
body; the palms of both
hands face each other as
if holding a ball. To-
gether with the body
(7) and arm movement, pull
left foot to the right
without touching the
(8) ground. Look at the
right hand. Take an
arched step left, while
(9) both arms pull away
from each other in an arclike movement.

The left hand moves forward and up, and the right han
(10) moves down somewhat to the side of the hips. Eyes foll
left hand up to 9 o'clock. Body turns somewhat diagona
the direction 10 o'clock.

(11) Prepare for an arched step to the right. Shift weight c
pletely to the left foot, placing the foot on its ball, whil
suming the *ball-holding position* with arms to the left. Tu
(12) body to 8 o'clock. Without breaking stride or touching
ground, pull right foot in rounded movement. Take a
(13) arched step to the right, first setting foot down with the
while pulling hands apart like (7) to (9); right hand mov
(14) left hand makes a rounded movement down. Eyes are o
right hand until it reaches 9 o'clock.

(15) Continue as in (10) to (14), just reverse *left* and *right*.
ing the mane" within each sequence takes place three ti
(19) altogether: to the right, to the left, to the right.

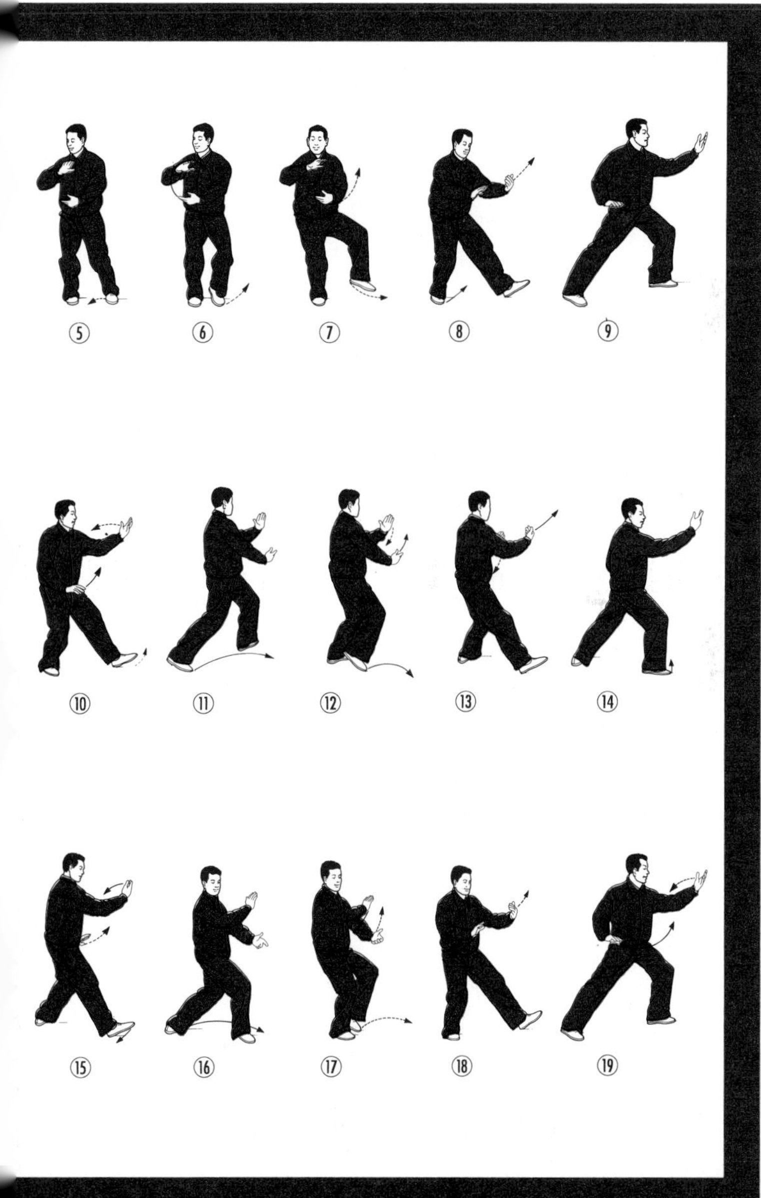
⑤
⑥
⑦
⑧
⑨
⑩
⑪
⑫
⑬
⑭
⑮
⑯
⑰
⑱
⑲

Stork Spreading Its Wings

20 With the last arched step, turn the body slightly to 8 o'clock; the weight is on the left foot, and the right foot is pulled towards the left by half the distance. At the same time, arms and hands move into the *ball-holding position* at the left of the body; body is turned to 8 o'clock.

21 Weight is shifted back to the right foot. During this stepping back, the body automatically turns to the right and is at the 10 o'clock position. While the body is rotating, the arms pull away from each other in arclike movements—left hand is moving down to the left, right arm moving up until it is opposite the forehead (palm facing forehead). Eyes follow the right hand.

Starting Position → 9 o'clock

22 While the hands are moving apart, the left foot—which is carrying no weight—takes a step (about 4–5 cm, or 2 inches) forward and—with leg slightly bent—lets the toes only touch the ground (see "Empty Step," page 71). In the end position, the eyes are facing 9 o'clock.

Note: There's a smooth, flowing transition between the end position of "Parting the Horse's Mane" and the beginning of "Stork Spreading Its Wings." Shifting of the weight to the back leg must be coordinated with the upward movement of the right arm. The upper body must not lean back!

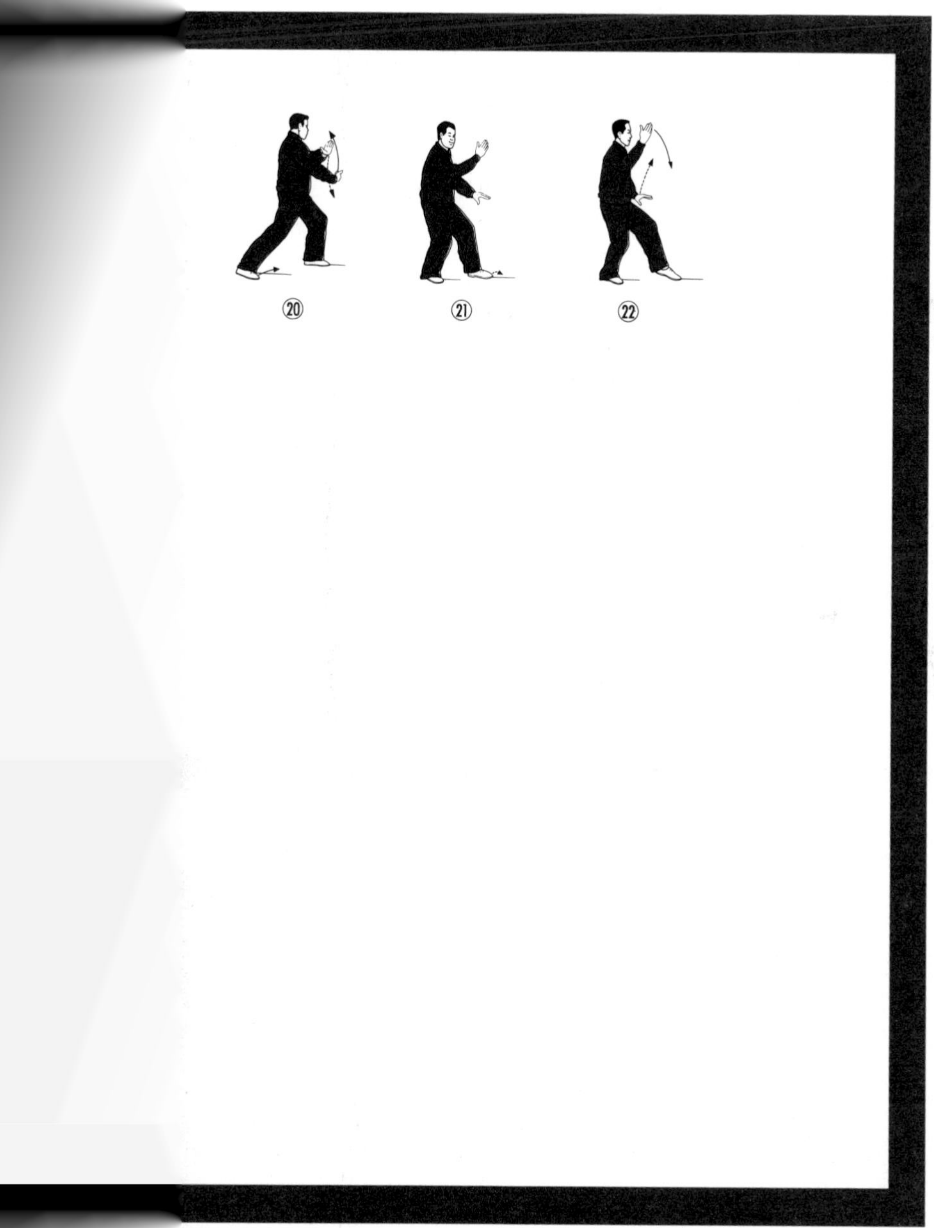
⑳
㉑
㉒

Brushing Your Knees & Stepping

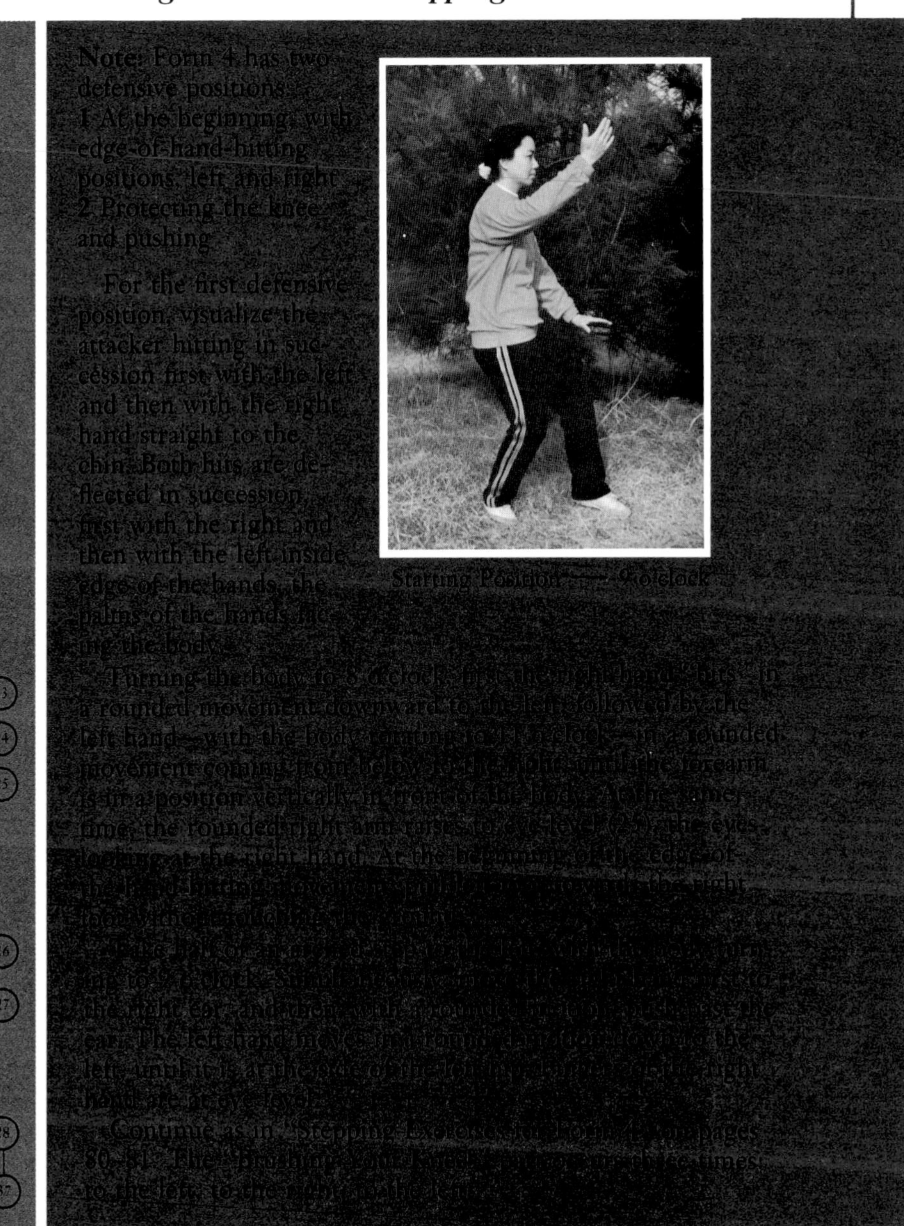

Starting Position ——— 9 o'clock

Note: Form 4 has two defensive positions:
1 At the beginning: with edge-of-hand-hitting positions, left and right
2 Protecting the knee and pushing

For the first defensive position, visualize the attacker hitting in succession first with the left and then with the right hand straight to the chin. Both hits are deflected in succession, first with the right and then with the left inside edge of the hands, the palms of the hands facing the body.

Turning the body to 8 o'clock, first the right hand "hits" in
23 a rounded movement downward to the left followed by the
24 left hand—with the body turning to 11 o'clock—in a rounded
25 movement coming from below to the right until the forearm
is in a position vertically in front of the body. At the same
time, the rounded right arm rises to eye level (25), the eyes
looking at the right hand. At the beginning of the edge-of-
the-hand-hitting movement, pull [illegible] towards the right
foot without touching the ground.
26 Take half of a [illegible] step [illegible] with the body turn-
27 ing to 9 o'clock. Simultaneously [illegible] the right hand [illegible] to
the right ear, and then with a rounded motion pushes past the
ear. The left hand moves in a rounded motion down to the
left until it is at the side of the left hip [illegible] of the right
hand are at eye level.
28 Continue as in "Stepping Exercises for Form 4" on pages
80–81. The "Brushing Your Knees" [illegible] three times:
37 to the left, to the right, to the left.

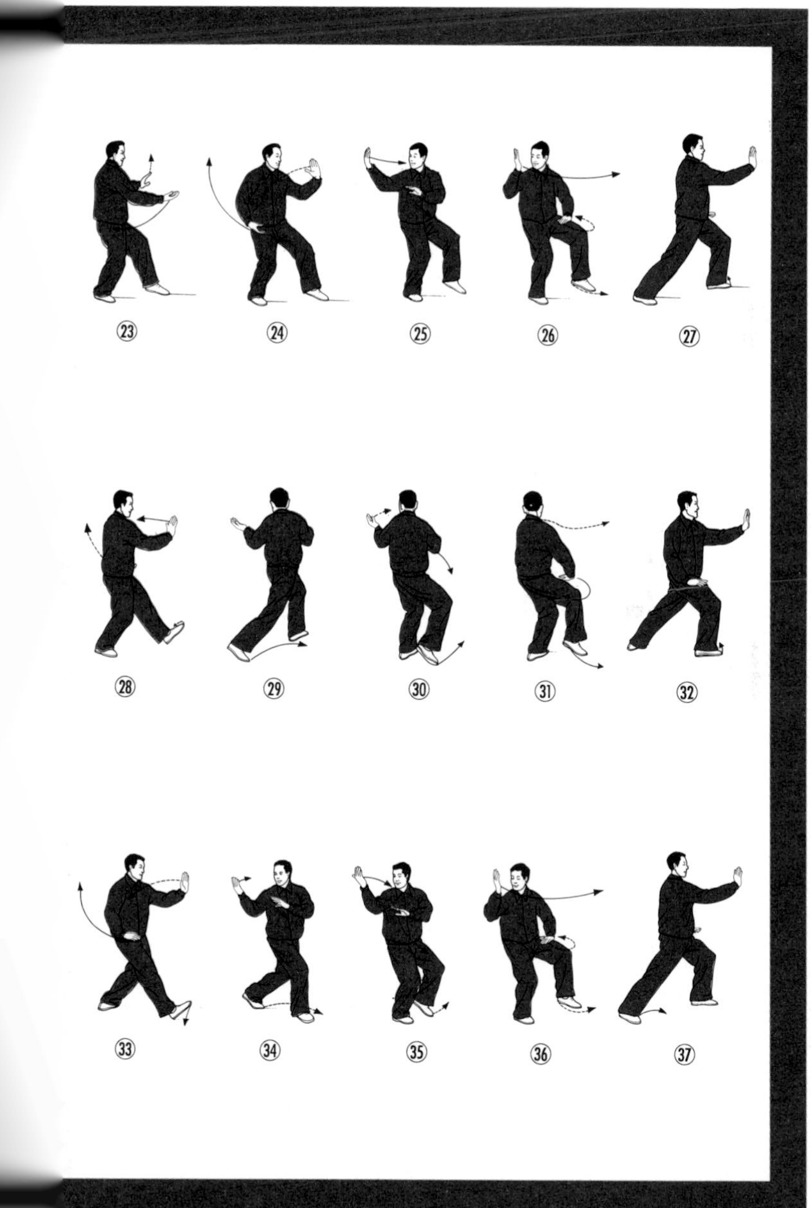
23
24
25
26
27
28
29
30
31
32
33
34
35
36
37

Playing the Pipa

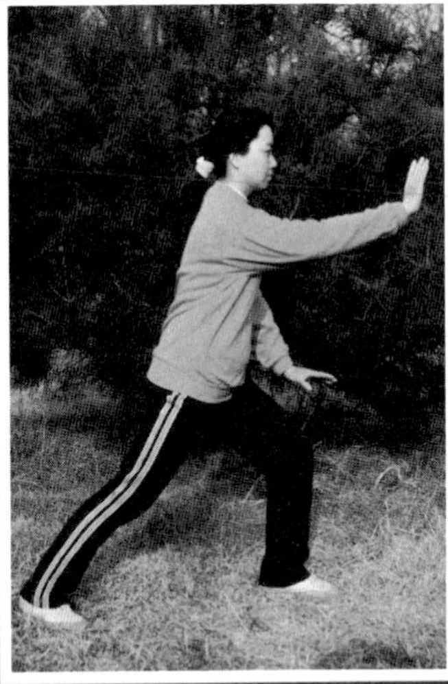

Starting Position ⟶ 9 o'clock

First perform the same
sequence of steps as in
Form 3, with the last
rounded step rotating
the body slightly to the
38 left to 8 o'clock—with
the full weight on the
left foot, while the right
foot moves to the left by
half the distance.

39 Shift the total weight
back to the right foot.

40 While stepping back,
the body automatically
rotates to the right to 10
o'clock. Along with step-
ping back, bend the left
arm slightly into an arc,
moving the arm up to eye level (palm facing out). The right
hand moves to the right with the rotation of the body, until it
is on the same level with the left elbow. The palm of the
right hand faces the left elbow. With the arm movement, lift
the left foot forward and set it on the ground with the heel
only (see "The Empty Step," on page 71). Look towards 9
o'clock.

Note: Smoothly coordinate the shifting of the weight while stepping back with the raising of the left hand.

The *pipa* is a Chinese musical instrument.

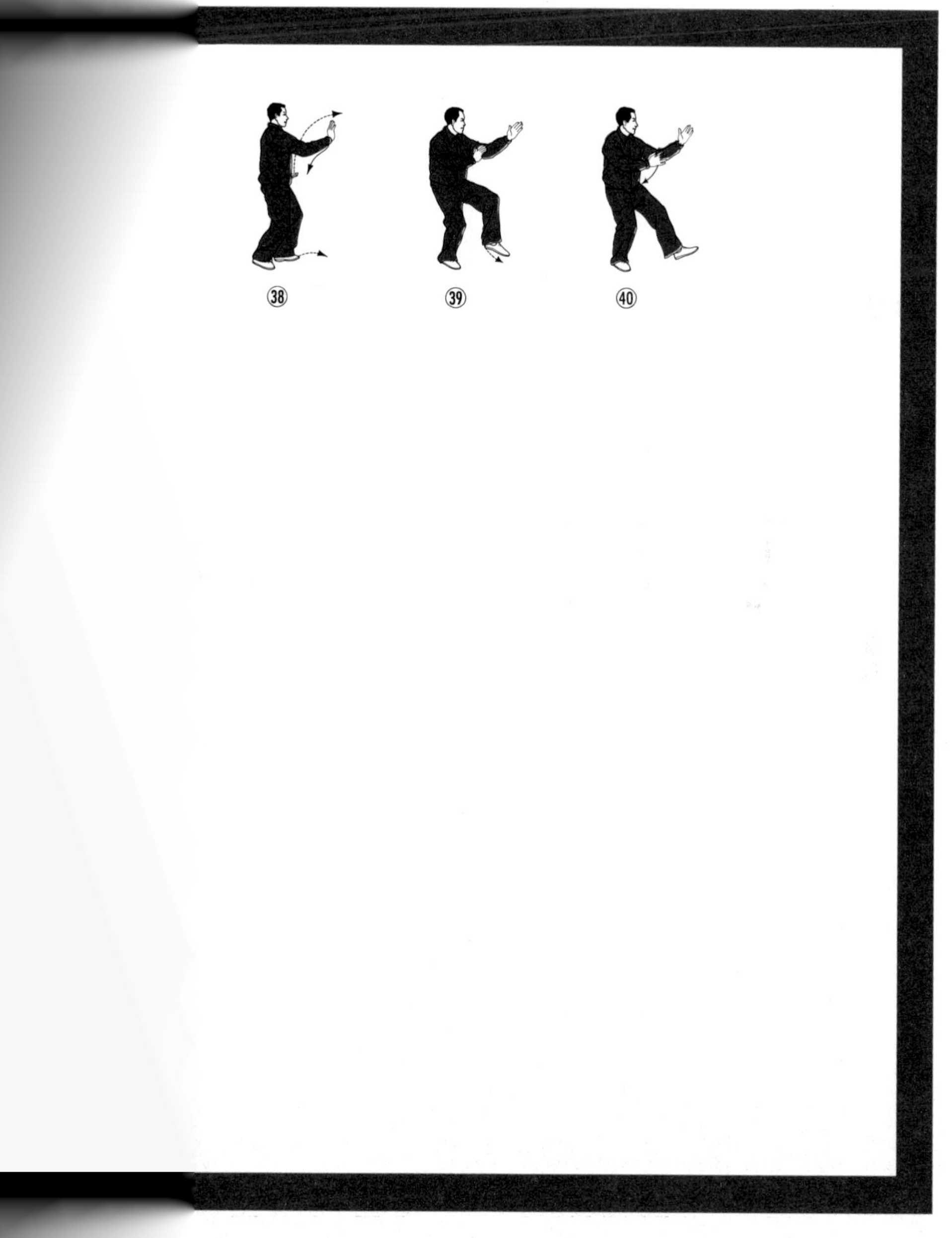
38
39
40

Fending Off the Monkey

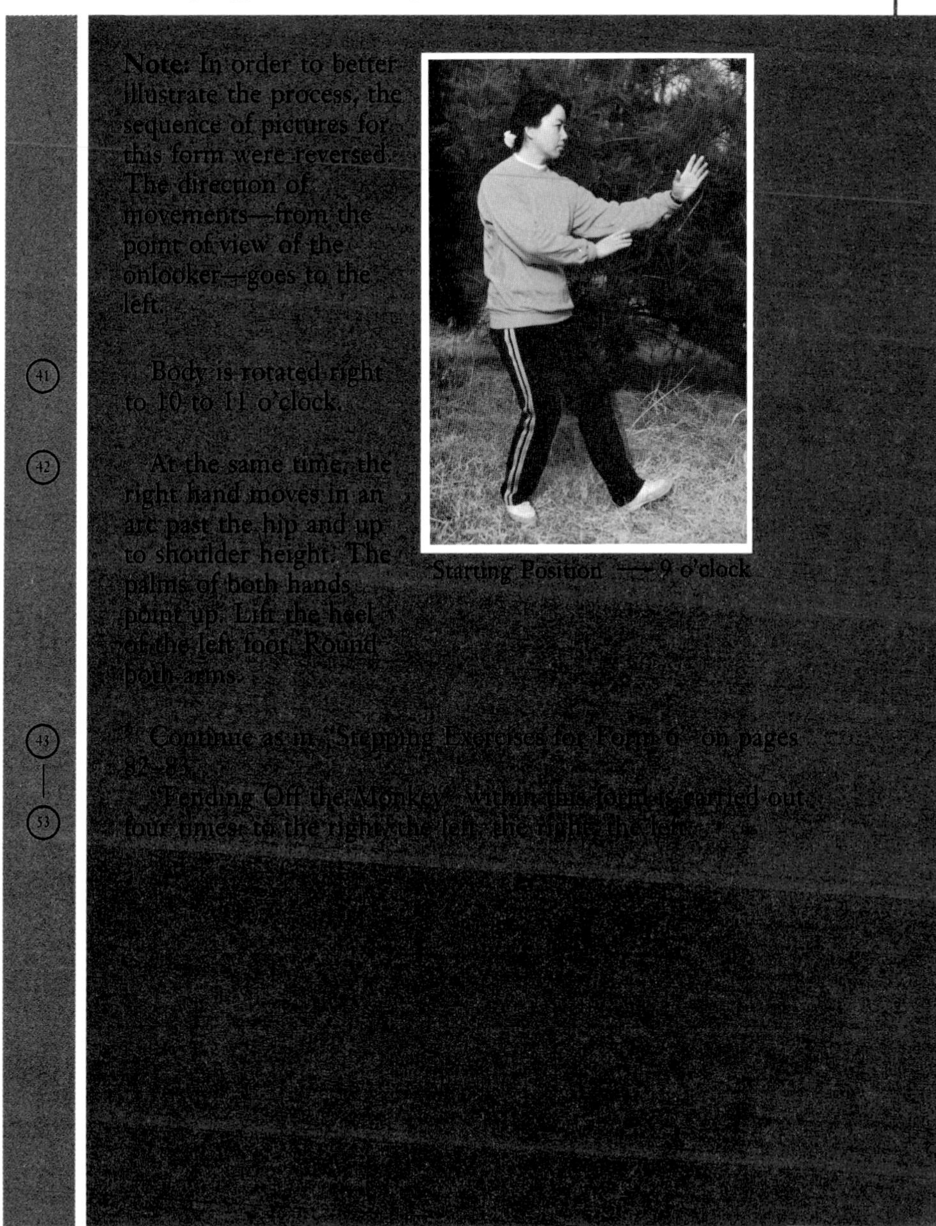

Note: In order to better illustrate the process, the sequence of pictures for this form were reversed. The direction of movements—from the point of view of the onlooker—goes to the left.

Starting Position → 9 o'clock

41 Body is rotated right to 10 to 11 o'clock.

42 At the same time, the right hand moves in an arc past the hip and up to shoulder height. The palms of both hands point up. Lift the heel of the left foot. Round both arms.

43–53 Continue as in "Stepping Exercises for Form 6" on pages 82–83.

"Fending Off the Monkey" within this form is carried out four times: to the right, the left, the right, the left.

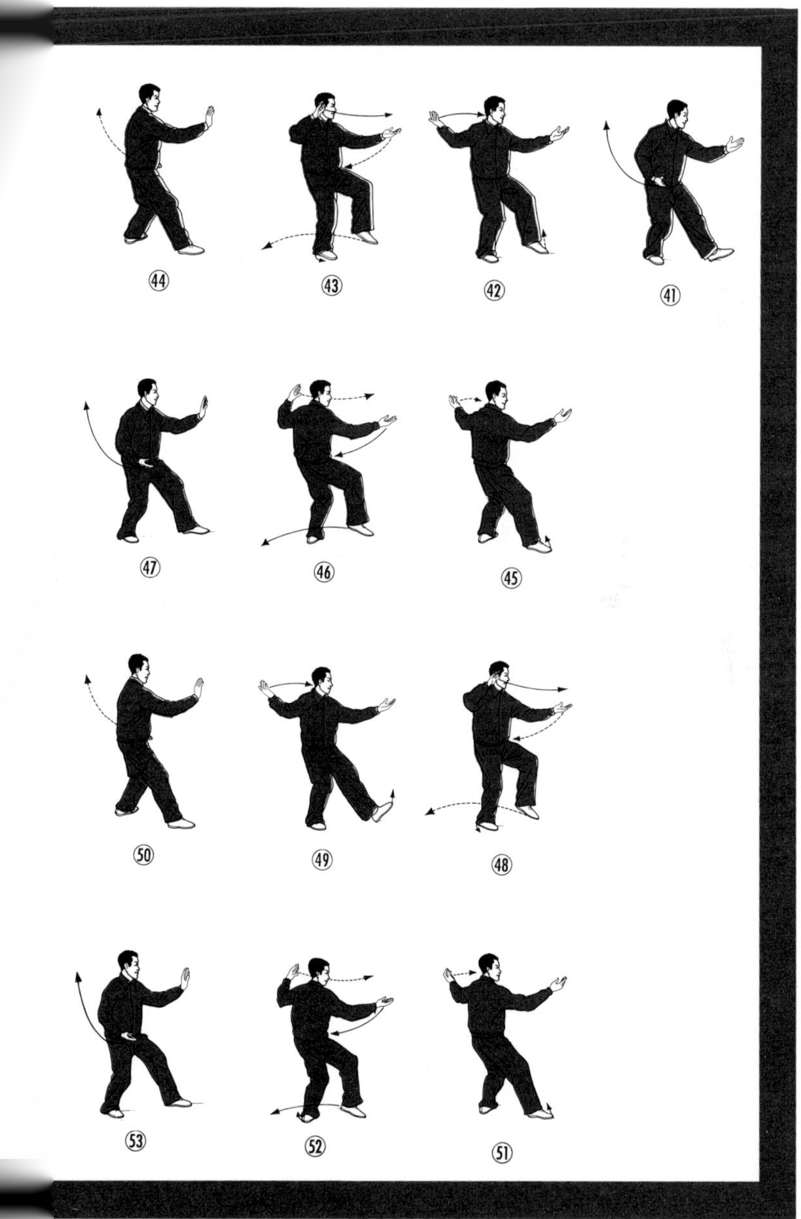
44
43
42
41
47
46
45
50
49
48
53
52
51

Grasping the Sparrow's Tail—Left & Right

Forms 7 and 8 consist of two identical parts that are carried out to the left and then to the right.

1 Peng movement—defense forward and up, picture series (56) to (58) and (70) to (72) respectively.

2 Lu movement—moving back and pulling, picture series (58) to (60) and (72) to (74) respectively.

3 Ji movement—pushing forward, picture series [illegible] to (78) and (74) to (76), respectively.

4 An movement—pushing, picture series (63) to (66) and (76) to (80) respectively.

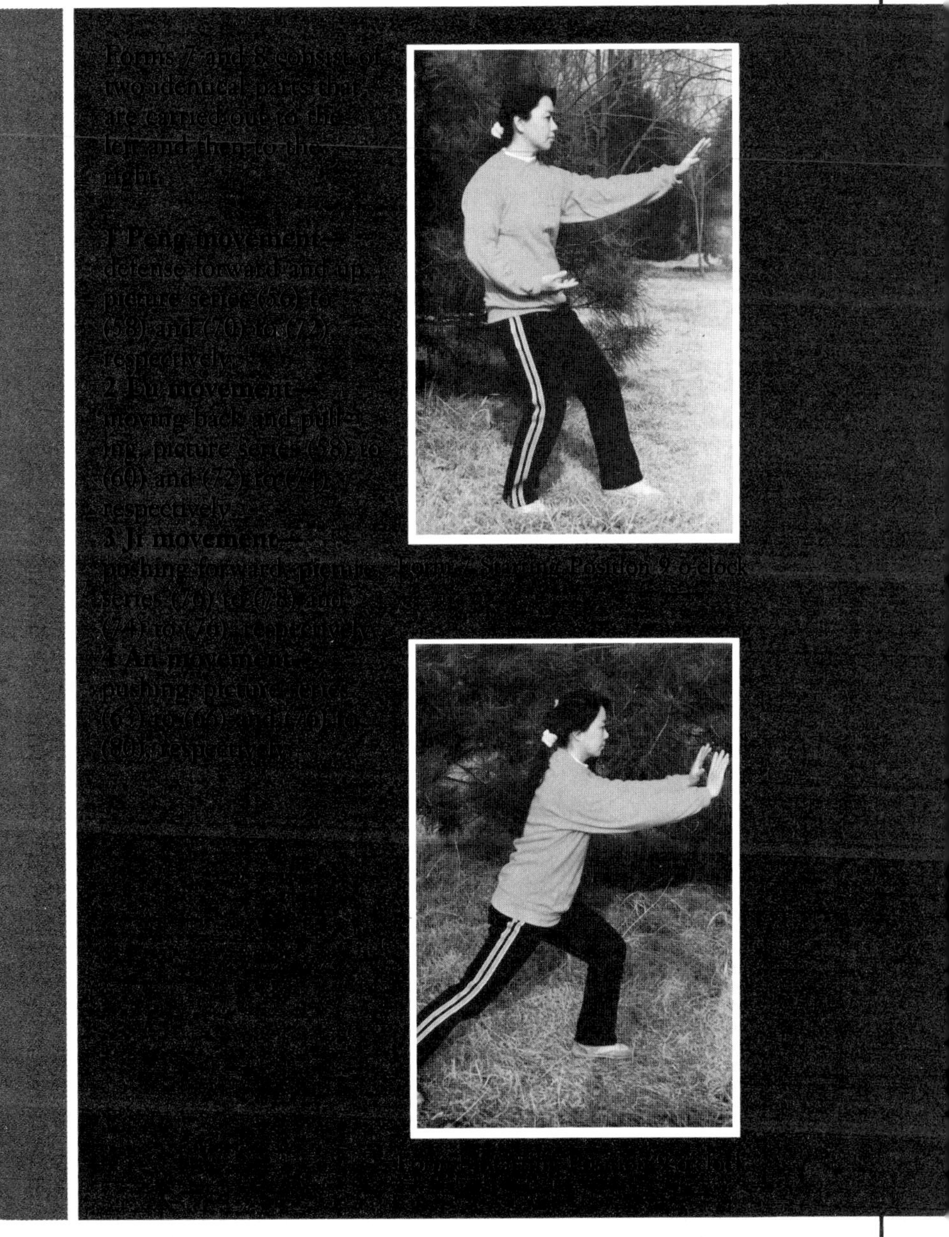

Form 7 Starting Position 9 o'clock

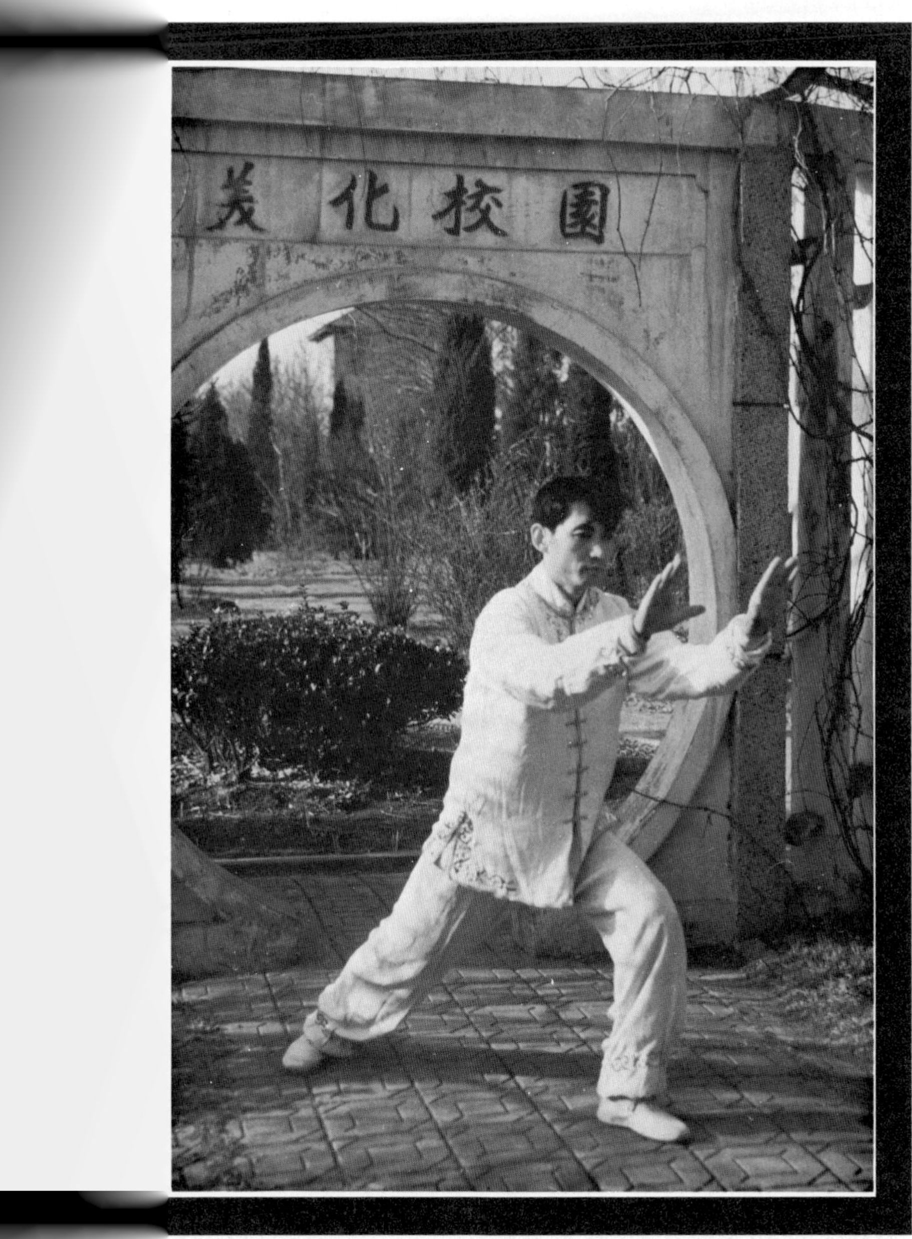
美化校園

Grasping the Sparrow's Tail—Left

Assume **starting position** (see page 104, top photo): Shift
weight to the right foot; left foot touches the ground with the
toes. Rotate body to the right to 11 o'clock. Move right hand
and arm in an arc diagonally up and then down in facing the
54 chest (55), while the left then moves in an arc down to
form—together with the right hand—the *holding-ball position*
56 (56). At the same time, pull the left foot to the right without
touching the ground. This position (56) is the starting point
for the first part of the form.

1. Peng movement: With an arched step to the left, pull
the right hand as in Form 2 ("Parting Horse's Mane") in an
57 arc down to hip level, while the left forearm—different from
Form 2—moves at a right angle in an arc forward and up un-
58 til level with the chest, harmoniously coordinating it with the
rotation of the body and the shifting of the weight. Position
(58) is the starting point for the second part of the form.

2. Lu movement: This starts with a slight rotation of the
body to 8 o'clock (not pictured). While the body rotates to
58 the left, hands are rotating to face each other, the right hand
moving towards the left. Both hands—while shifting the
59 weight to the right leg and rotating the body to 10 to 11
o'clock—move in an arc down to the right at hip level.

Position (59) is the starting point for the third part of the
form.

3. Ji movement: Preceded by a small reaching-back move-
59 ment, move the right hand towards the left; both hands cross
at the wrists and are pushed forward and out. Keep arms
62 rounded—not straight. When pushing forward, shift the
weight again to the left leg. Position (62) is the starting point
for the fourth part of the form.

62 **4. An movement:** At the conclusion of the ji movement,
turn the hands so that they are crossed with the palms facing
down, the left hand below the right.

63 *—Please turn*

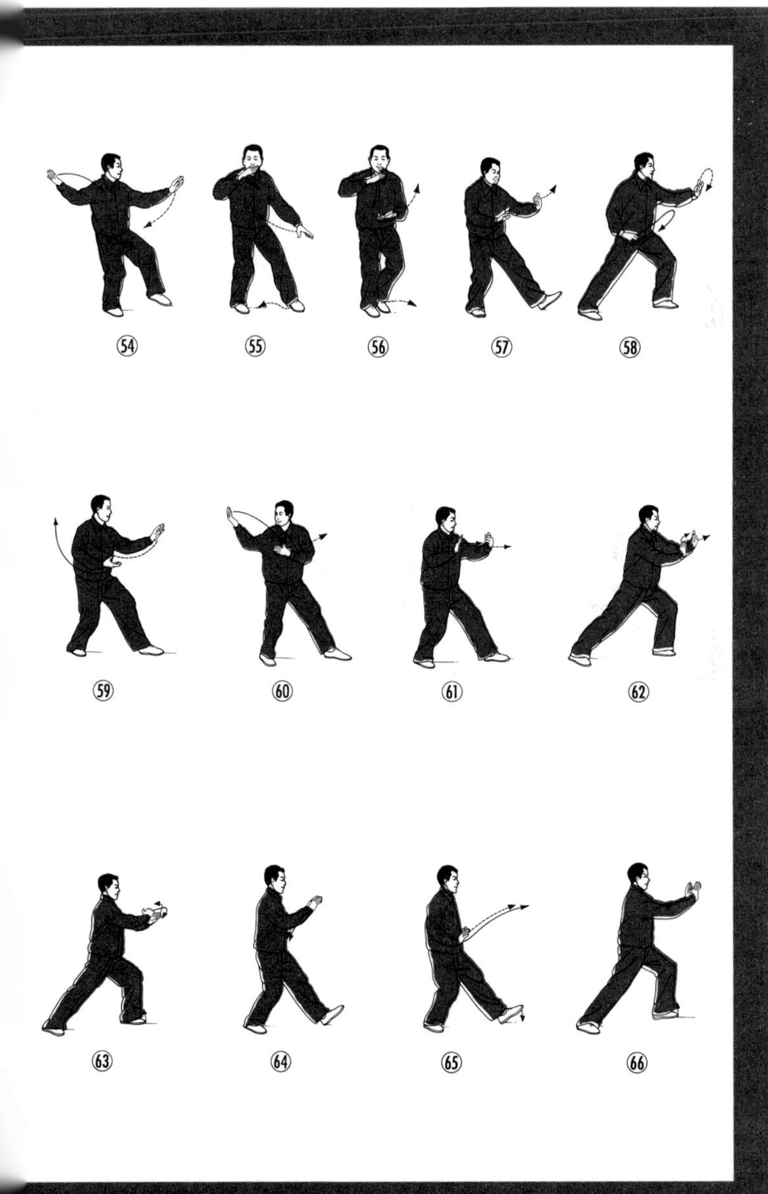

54
55
56
57
58
59
60
61
62
63
64
65
66

64 As the weight is shifted to the back right leg—the toes of the left foot raised slightly off the ground—the crossed hands
66 separate again and are pulled towards the body by the elbows. They are then—with a slight shift of the body's weight—pushed forward. Do not straighten your arms out in the end position of (66).

Note: The different parts of the form should flow easily into each other.

Grasping the Sparrow's Tail—Right

Assume **starting position** (see lower photo on page 104): Arch steps to the left. Left foot load about 70 percent; right foot about 30 percent.

67 Shift weight to the right foot, left foot rotates on the heel by 90 to 120° to the inside.

68 At the same time—with gently held, slightly rounded arms—the hands move with the upper body to the right.

69 Slowly bend arms, with right hand moving in an upward arc, and assume the *ball-holding position* in front of the right side of the body. While in the ball-holding position, the right
70 foot is pulled towards the left without the toes touching the ground.

71 Position (70) is the starting point for the first part of the form, the Peng. Follow the same sequence of movements as
80 in (56) through (66), but exchange *left* for *right*.

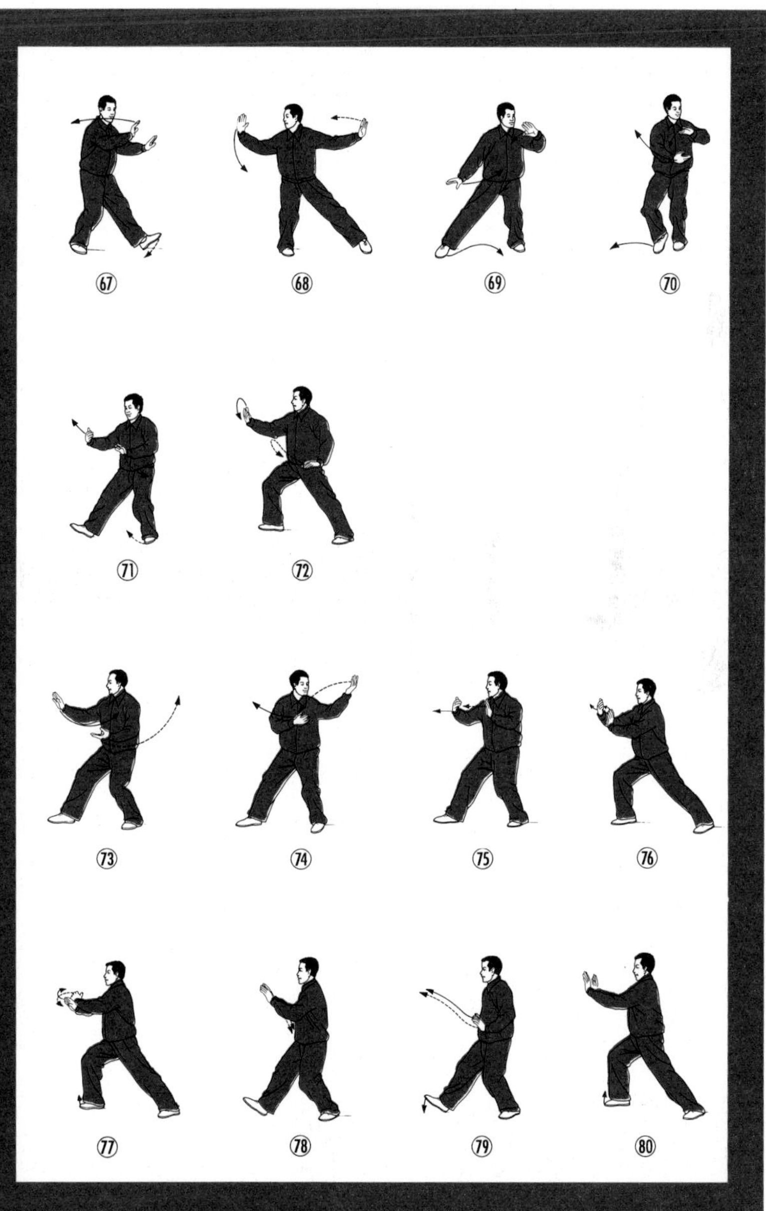
67
68
69
70
71
72
73
74
75
76
77
78
79
80

Simple Whip

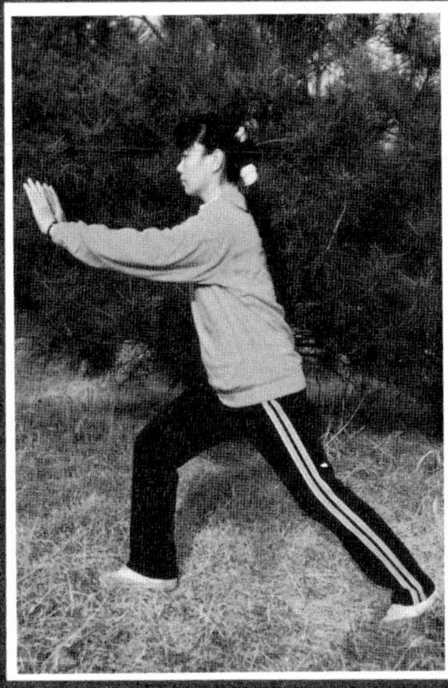

Starting Position ⟶ 3 o'clock

(81)–(82) Shift weight back to the left leg. While rotating the body to about 11 o'clock, turn the right foot—on its heel—by about 100 to 110° inside to the right. At the same time, the right hand moves in an arc (81) and then up again (82). The downward movement is coordinated with the rotation of the foot. Similarly, but in the opposite direction of the right hand, the left hand makes a circular downward movement.

(83)–(84) Together with the right hand moving up (body is positioned at 11 o'clock) (82), the weight is shifted again to the right leg and the left foot is pulled to the right foot. The right hand moves, at eye level, in front of the face (with the palm pointing to the body); then the left palm is turned over, relaxing the wrist and forming a *dropped hand* (see page 64), while the right arm is bent at about 120° in the direction of the movement at 9 o'clock.

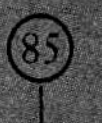

(85)–(86) In coordination with the arched step to the left, the body turns to 10 o'clock, allowing the rounded left arm to move with the turn. Along with shifting the weight to the left foot and pushing the body forward, the left hand is rotated to the outside at 9 o'clock.

Note: The right arm is not stretched out completely when the hand is in the dropped position. The dropped hand is slightly above shoulder level. The left arm is not pushed forward with the movement of the body.

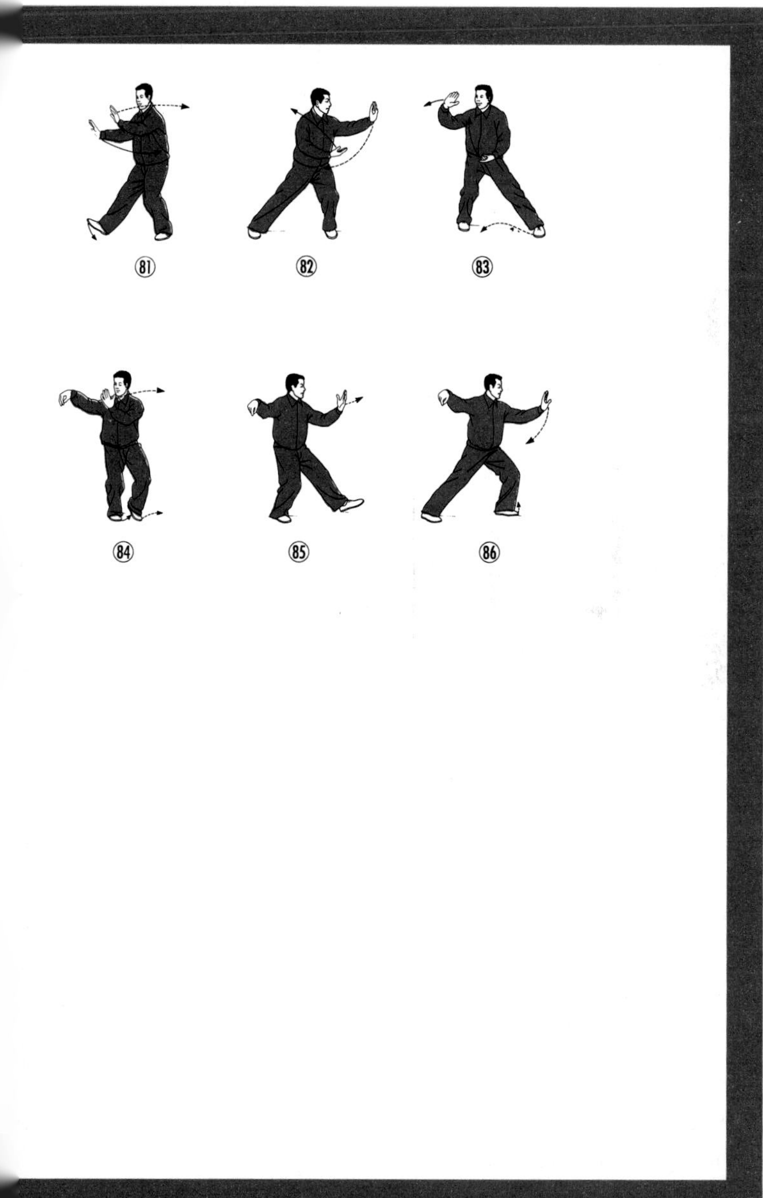
81
82
83
84
85
86

Moving Hands Like Clouds

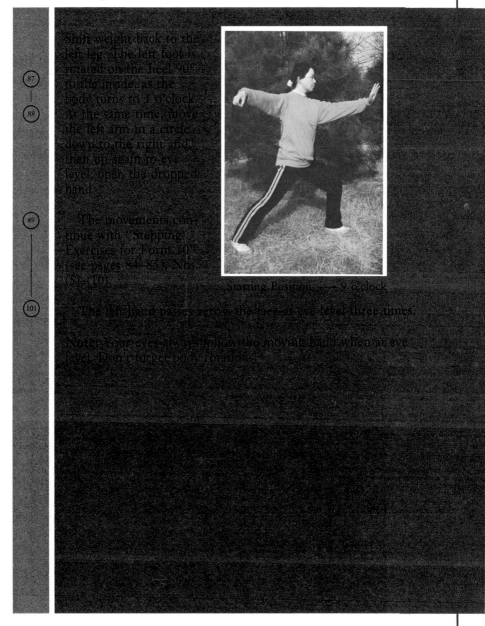

(87)–(88) Shift weight back to the left leg. The left foot is rotated on the heel 90° to the inside, as the body turns to 1 o'clock. At the same time, move the left arm in a circle down to the right and, then up again to eye level; open the dropped hand.

(89)–(101) The movements continue with "Stepping Exercises for Form 10" (see pages 84–85), Nos. (5)–(10).

Starting Position ⟶ 9 o'clock

The left hand passes across the face at eye level three times.

Note: Your eyes always follow the moving hand when at eye level. Don't forget body rotations!

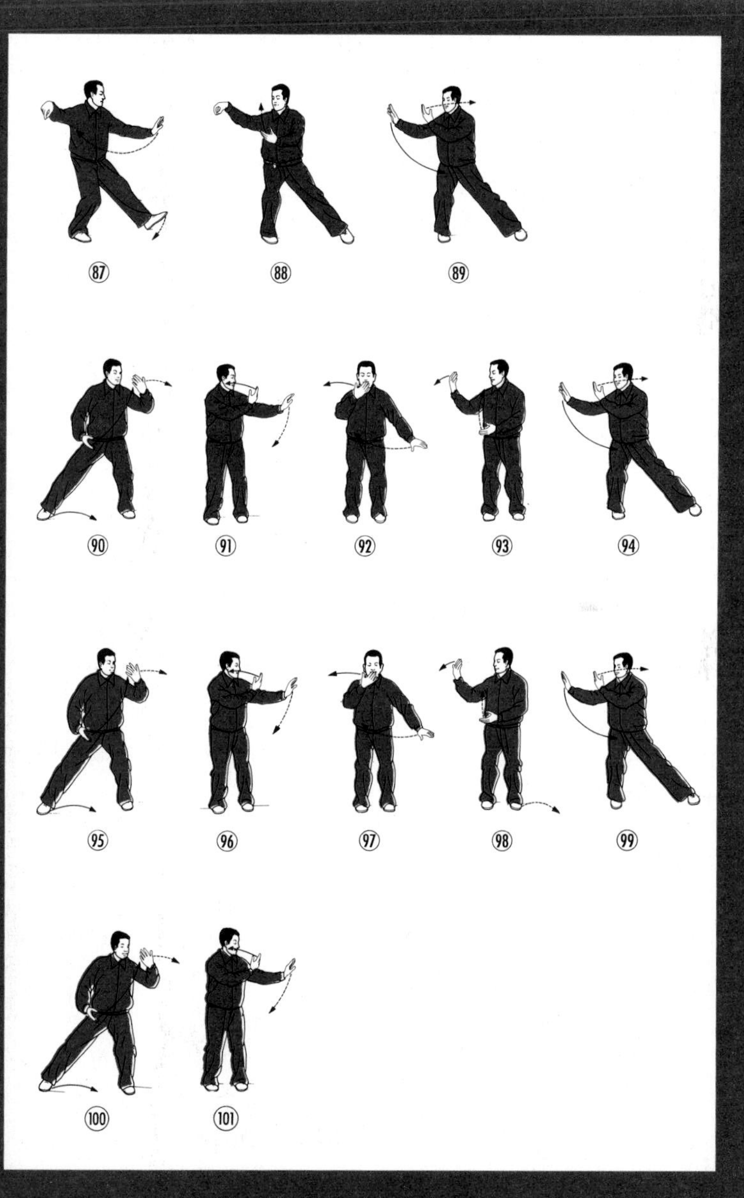
87
88
89
90
91
92
93
94
95
96
97
98
99
100
101

Simple Whip

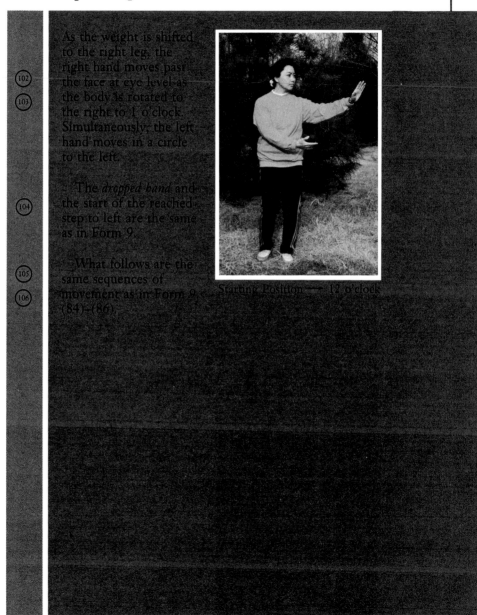

As the weight is shifted
to the right leg, the
right hand moves past
(102) the face at eye level as
(103) the body is rotated to
the right to 1 o'clock.
Simultaneously, the left
hand moves in a circle
to the left.

The *dropped hand* and
(104) the start of the reached
step to left are the same
as in Form 9.

(105) What follows are the
same sequences of
(106) movement as in Form 9
(84)–(86).

Starting Position → 12 o'clock

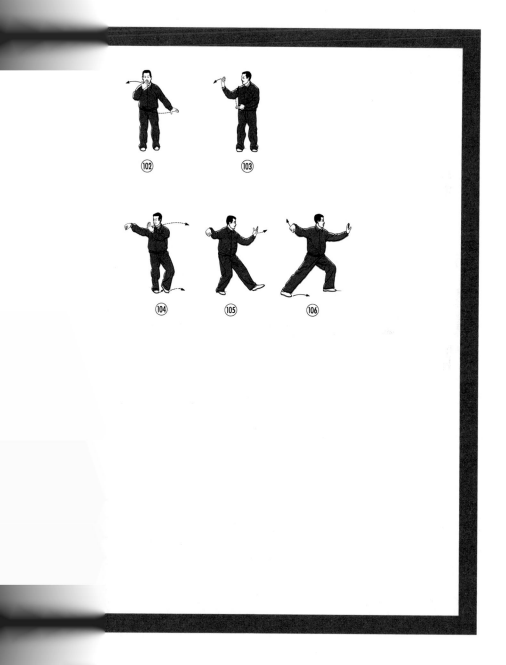
102
103
104
105
106

Patting the Horse's Neck While Riding

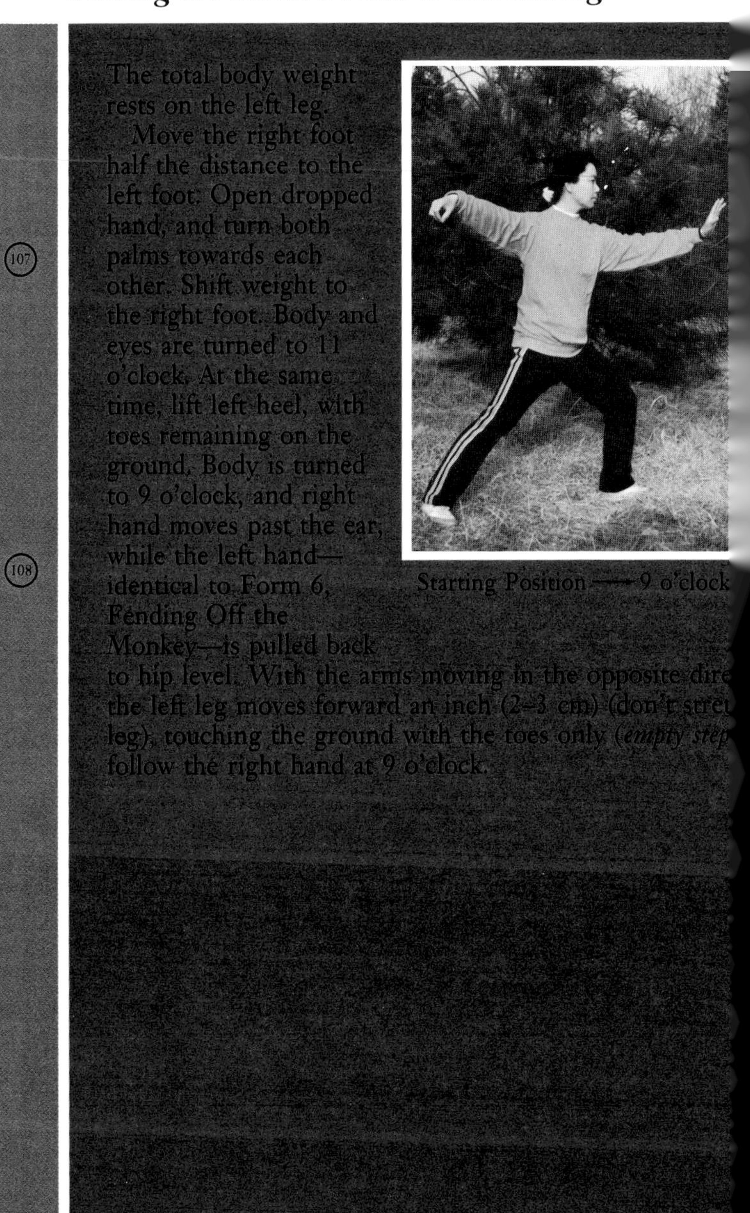

Starting Position —— 9 o'clock

The total body weight rests on the left leg.

Move the right foot half the distance to the left foot. Open dropped hand, and turn both
107 palms towards each other. Shift weight to the right foot. Body and eyes are turned to 11 o'clock. At the same time, lift left heel, with toes remaining on the ground. Body is turned to 9 o'clock, and right hand moves past the ear, while the left hand—
108 identical to Form 6, Fending Off the Monkey—is pulled back to hip level. With the arms moving in the opposite dire the left leg moves forward an inch (2–3 cm) (don't stret leg), touching the ground with the toes only (*empty step* follow the right hand at 9 o'clock.

107
108

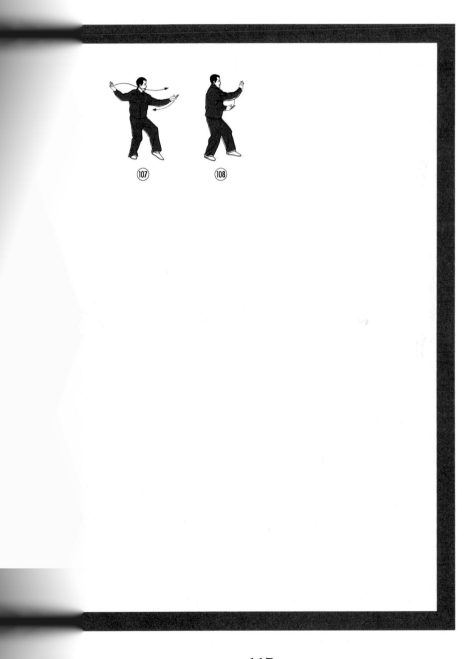

Right Heel Kick

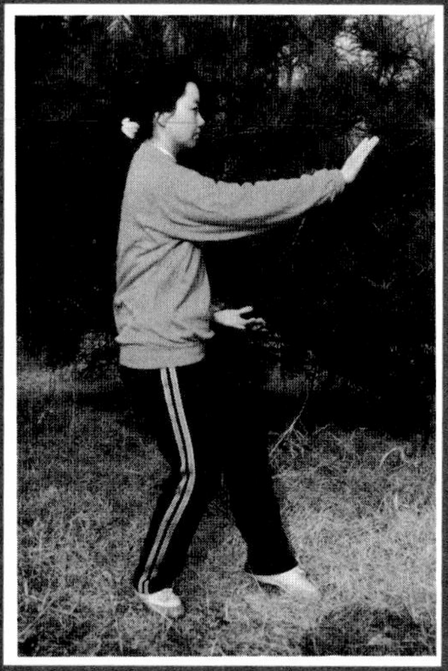

Rotate body to 8
o'clock, while the left
109 hand crosses above the
right hand at the wrists;
at the same time, lift the
111 left leg and place the
foot—heel first—on the
ground to the left about
30° from the direction
of the movement, at 9
o'clock. Separate hands
and move them down in
a circle as if you were
caressing a ball.

Starting Position — 9 o'clock

Both hands, again,
cross at the wrists, as the
112 circular movements are
performed. The right
hand is on the outside, and palms of both hands face the
body. At the same time, pull the right leg towards the left
without touching the ground.

113 Separate hands, both arms moving to the side at shoulder
level and palms turned forward. Simultaneously, the right
knee is pulled up, and—coordinated with the stretching of the
114 arms—the right foot, at 10 o'clock, is raised for the *heel kick*,
as the toes are flexed. Eyes look to the right hand. Right arm
is parallel to the right leg.

Note: The kicking action and the separating of the hands/arms happens at the same time. Legs in (114) are at a 60° angle to each other. Try to avoid the body leaning back.

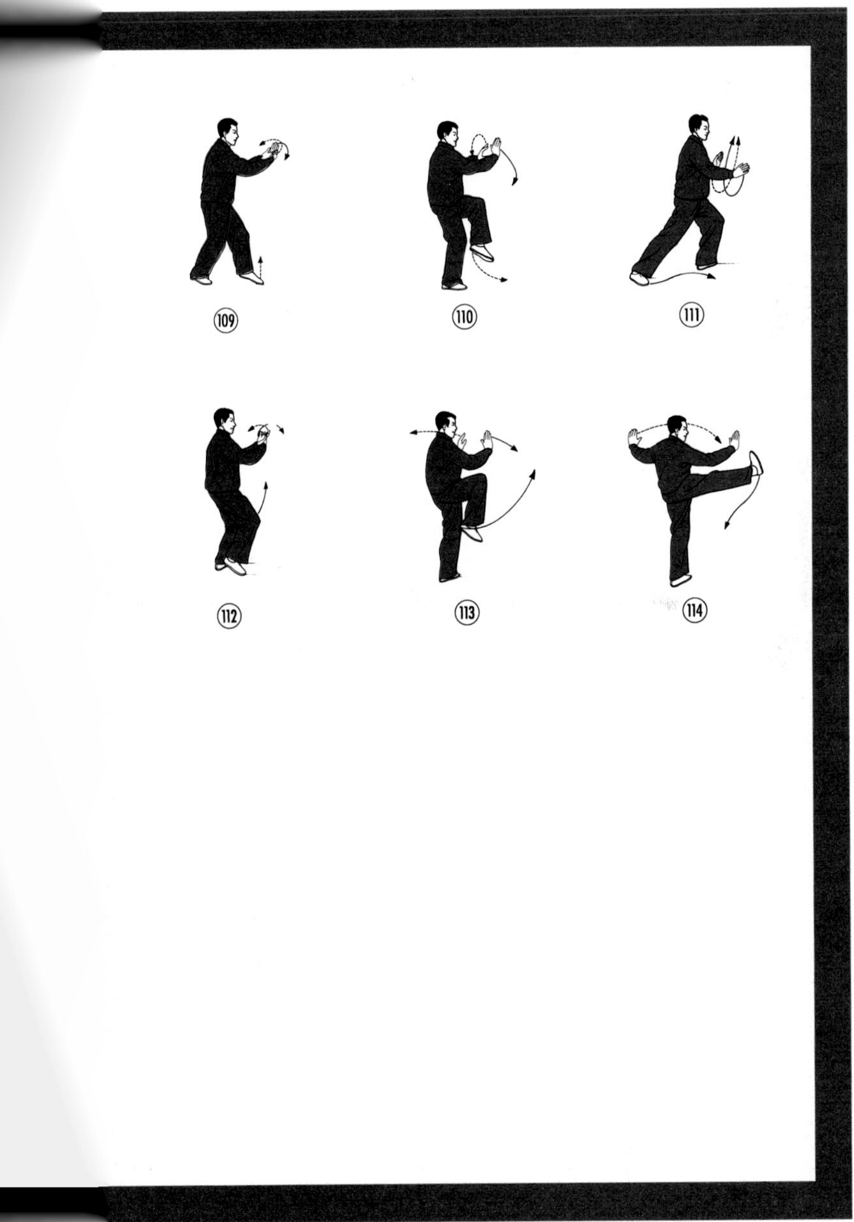
109
110
111
112
113
114

Hitting Your Opponent with Both Fists

115 At hip level, bend the right leg, while moving the left arm parallel to the right arm, turning the palms of both hands to face up.

116 Pull both hands in an arc down along each side of the right bent knee to hip level.

117 Gently bend the left leg, and set the right foot forward at 10 to 11 o'clock, while lowering the hands and forming fists.

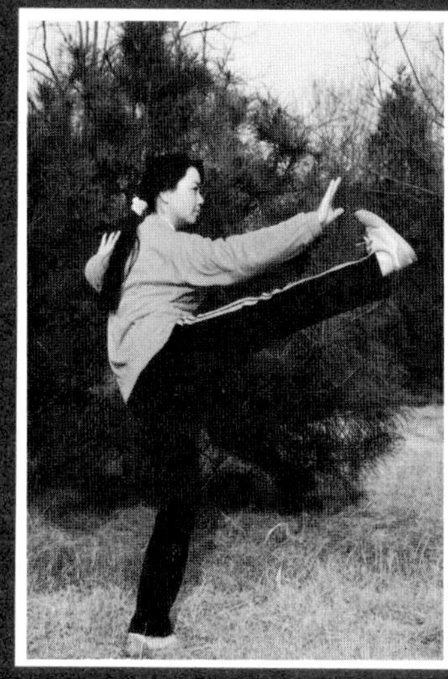

Starting Position → 10 o'clock

118 Similar to a pair of pliers, move fists sideways, forward, and up, while rotating the arms upward. This movement ends at eye level, where the distance of the fists is about the width of the head. Both fists are pointing towards the body. Shift weight to the right leg, as the fists are raised.

Note: Keep head straight. Shoulders and arms are relaxed, arms rounded. Do not clench your fists or round your back. Eyes in the end position are at 10 to 11 o'clock.

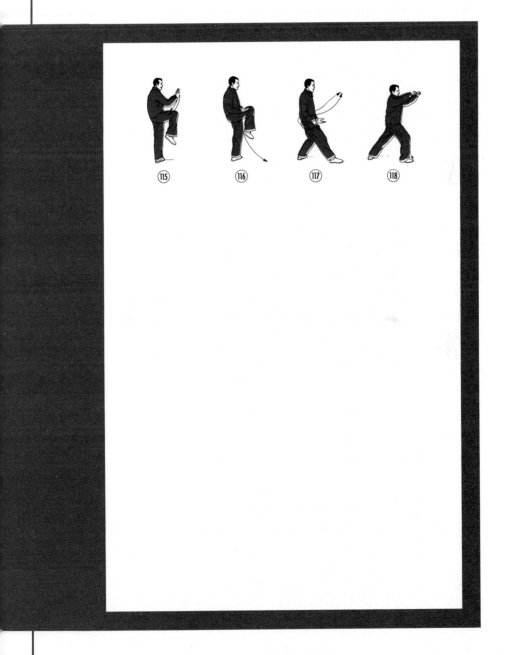
115
116
117
118

Left Heel Kick

(119)–(120) Shift weight to the left leg. While rotating the body to the left to 7 to 8 o'clock, rotate the heel of the right foot to the inside by about 90°. Arms and fists remain for now in the raised forward-pointing position (see photo at right), following the rotation of the body.

(120)–(121) Shift weight to the right leg and open fists.

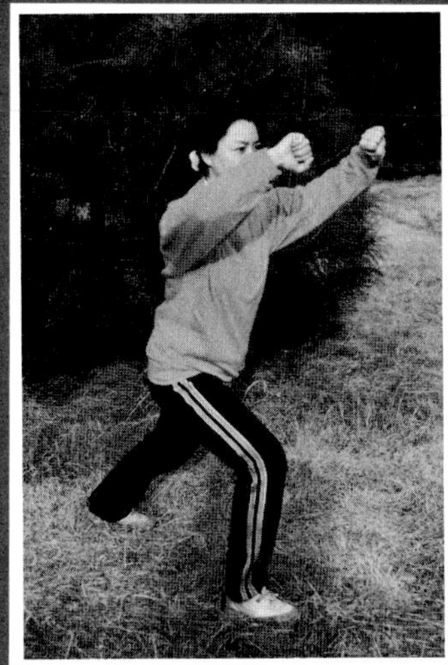

Starting Position —10–11 o'clock

(122)–(124) The rest of the movements are identical to Form 13 (112)–(114), except that *left* and *right* are reversed. As the left leg stretches, the body rotates to 5 to 6 o'clock. Eyes are looking at the left hand in the end position.

Note: All movements flow easily into one another. Reaching the end position does not mean that the flow of the movements comes to a halt. When hands cross each other, the left is on the outside.

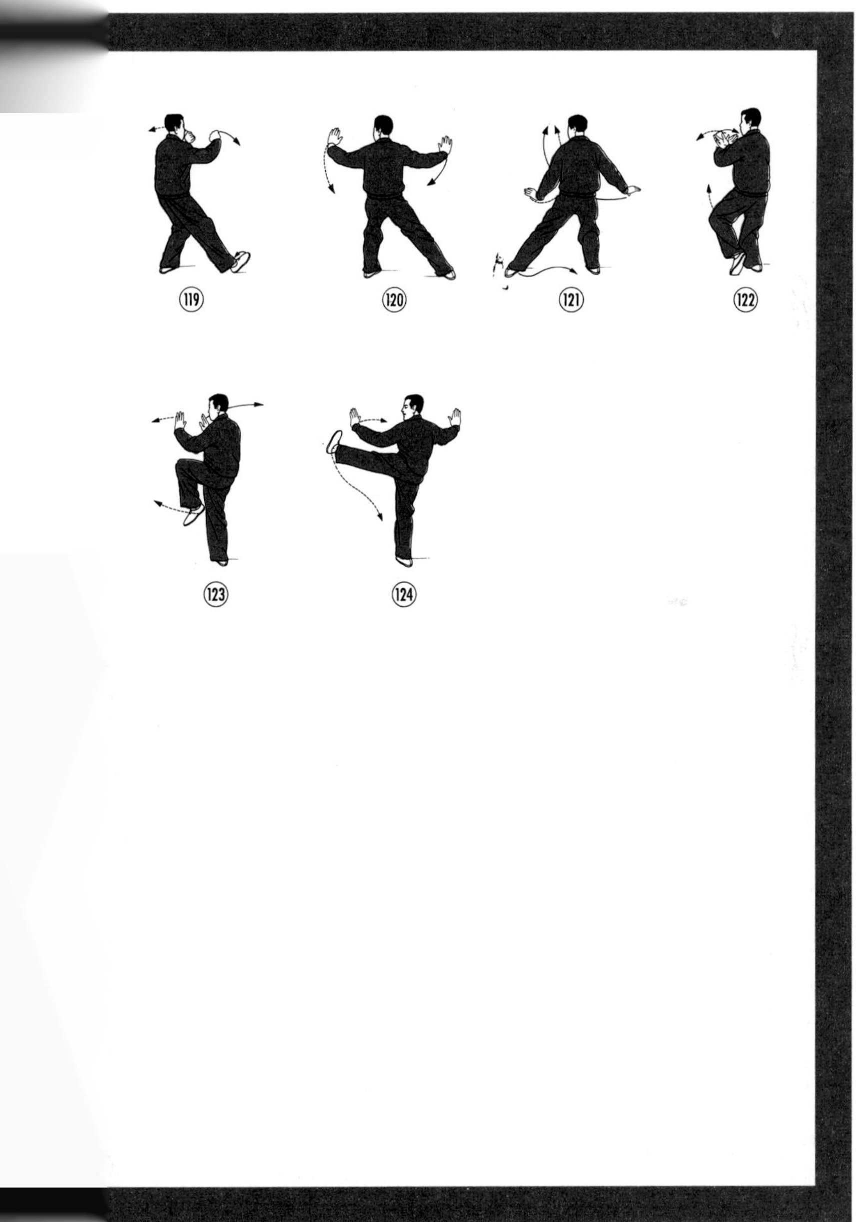
119
120
121
122
123
124

Crooked Whip—Left

Note: Forms 16 and 17 consist of two parts each that, for simplicity's sake, are combined under *one* name: Crooked Whip—Left & Right. They are also called Climbing Down & Standing on One Leg (Right or Left) and Rooster Standing on One Leg (Right or Left).

Starting Position → 5 o'clock

125—126 Bend left leg and rotate body to the right to 6 to 7 o'clock. The right hand changes to a *dropped hand*, while the left hand moves in a slight arc forward to chest level, palms of hands are pointing towards the body, eyes are looking to the dropped hand.

127—128 Bend right leg, lower the body, and bend body forward; the left foot—moved back the distance of one foot—extends out, sliding along the ground to 2 o'clock. The left hand moves down at the same time, palms facing the body, fingers pointing to 9 o'clock. While the left foot slides to the side, the left hand rotates 180° with fingers pointing to 5 o'clock. While the left foot is sliding, rotate it to face 2 to 3 o'clock (128).

129—131 Shift the weight in a flowing motion to the left leg; let the right leg follow and pull up the knee (131). While the left hand is lowered to hip level, the rotated dropped hand is pulled in a deep arc, opened, and moved upward (129). The edge of the hand is pointing to 3 o'clock.

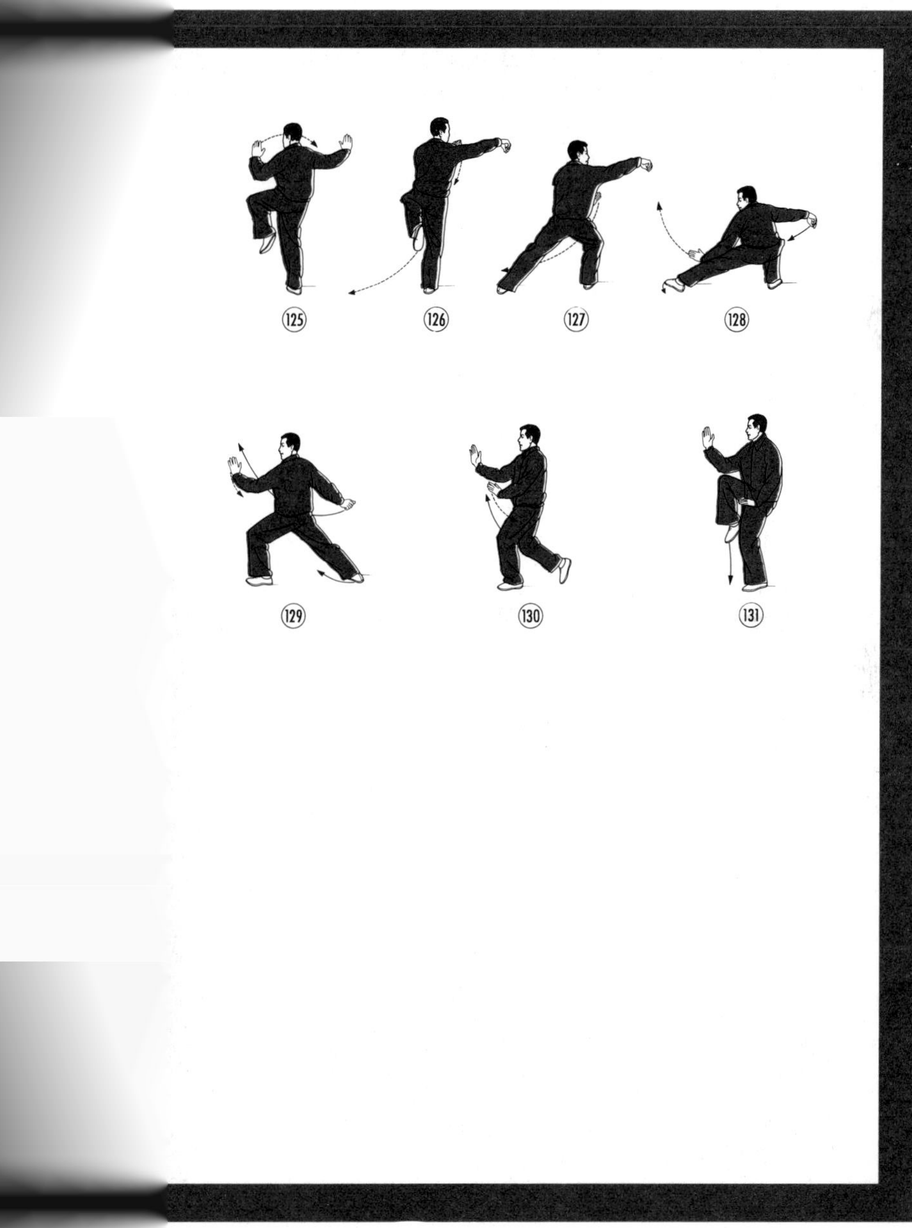
125
126
127
128
129
130
131

Crooked Whip—Right

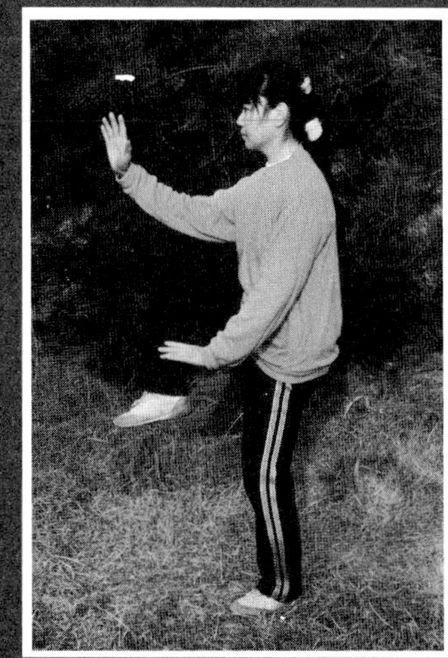

Starting Position → 3 o'clock

132–133 Lower the right leg; toes of the right foot at 1 o'clock are placed in front of the left foot. At the same time, the body rotates to the left to 12 o'clock, and the left arm is raised sideways to shoulder height (arm points to 10 to 11 o'clock), the wrist lowering to form a dropped hand. The right arm is moved in an arc in front of the left shoulder (133), the palms of the hands facing the body; the eyes look at the dropped hand.

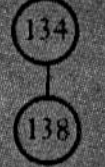

The following movements are identical to those of (127)–(131), except that *left* and *right* are reversed. In the end position, the body and the eyes are turned to 3 o'clock.

Note: Lowering the body, sliding, and raising the body again must be harmoniously coordinated with the arm/hand movements. The right and left hands must reach the end position at the same time.

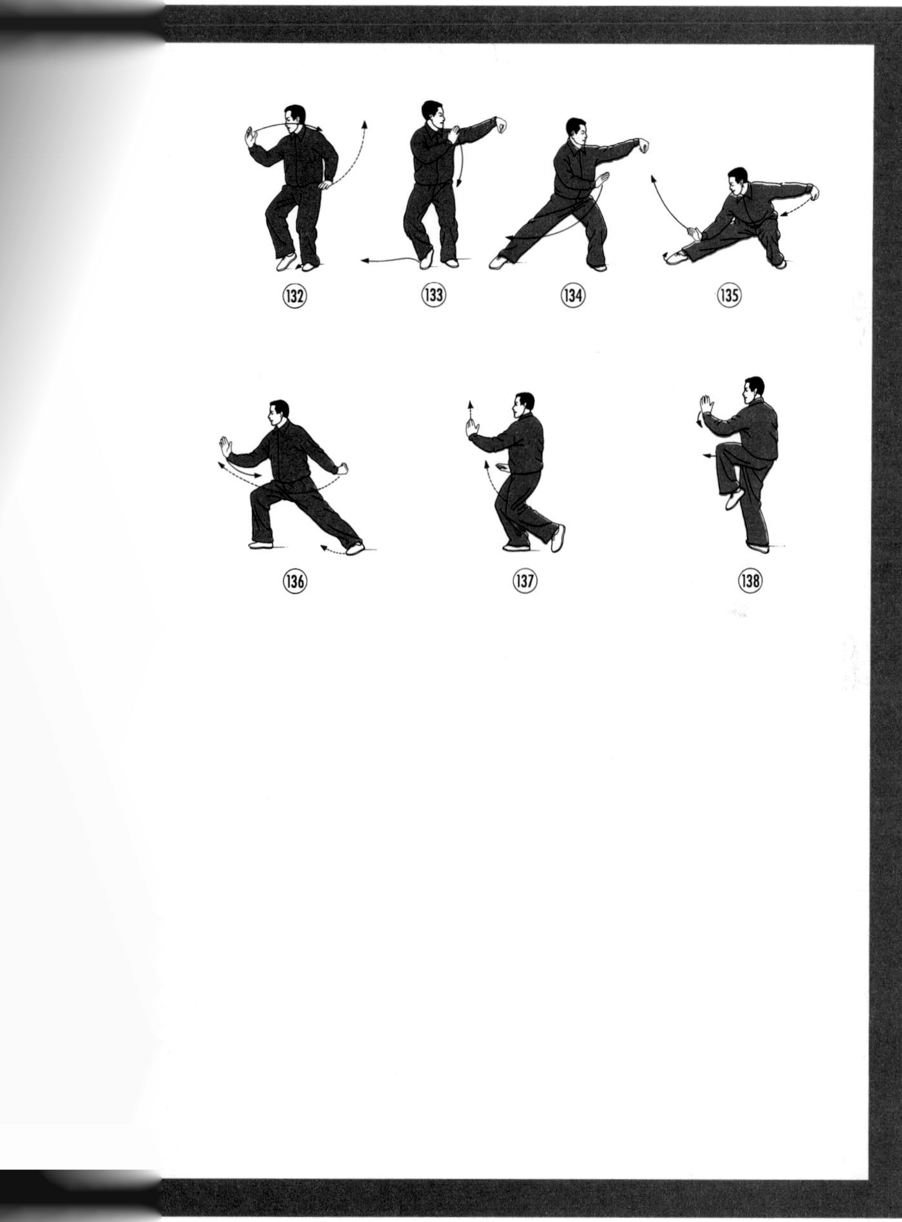
132
133
134
135
136
137
138

Throwing the Loom—Left & Right

139—140 Body is turned to 1 to 2 o'clock, and the left foot is placed with an arch-like motion 45° to the direction of the movement to the left. At the same time, both hands assume the *ball-holding position* in front of the right side of the chest, with the right hand below the left hand.

141 Pull the right foot next to the left (without touching the ground).

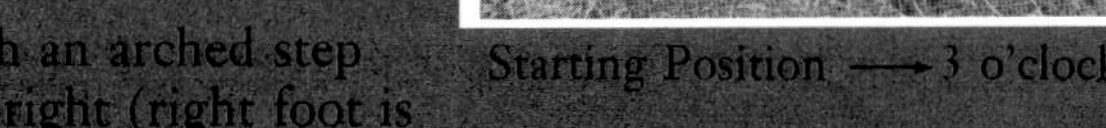

Starting Position ⟶ 3 o'clock

142—144 With an arched step to the right (right foot is at a 30° angle to the direction of the movement at 3 o'clock), the body also rotates to the right. At the same time, the right forearm moves in an arc upward and past the head, the head turning outward (back of the hand is in front of the forehead). With the upward movement of the right forearm and the shifting of the weight to the right leg, the left hand—in front of the left side of the chest—pushes up and forward at eye level. Eyes are on the left hand.

144 Shift weight back to the left leg, while lifting the toes of the right foot slightly off the ground. Slightly lower elbows; arms are relaxed (144).
145 Shift weight back fully to the right foot, pulling the left foot to the right foot and assuming the *ball-holding position* in front of the right side of the chest, right hand on top, body facing 4 o'clock (145).

146—149 While taking an arched step to the left (left foot at 3 o'clock), the sequence of movements continues with (141) to (144), except that *left* and *right* are reversed. Eyes are looking to 2 o'clock in the end position.

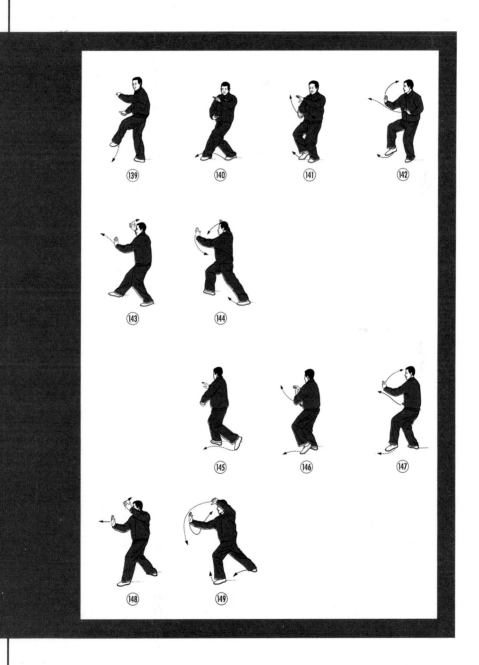
139
140
141
142
143
144
145
146
147
148
149

Needle at the Bottom of the Ocean

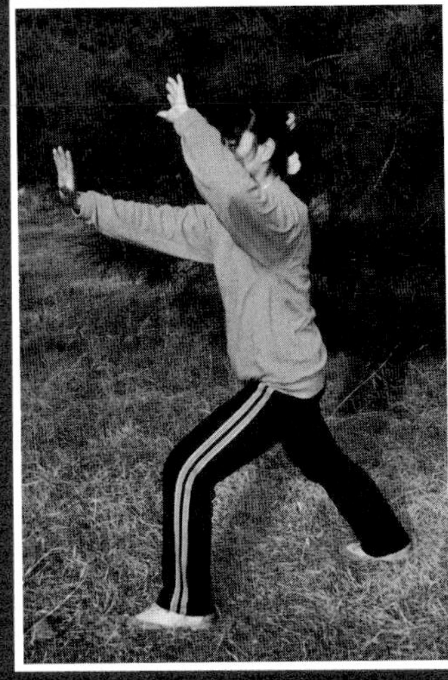

Starting Position — 2 o'clock

Pull the right foot half the distance to the left foot, shifting the full weight to the right foot. Rotate body to the right to 4 o'clock. Both hands move down in a looping motion (see (149)) and then upward again to head level; the right hand is slightly higher than the left.

Lift left leg slightly, pushing forward and
150 letting the toes (only)
touch the ground at
about 3 o'clock (*empty
step*, full weight on the
right foot). As the left
151 leg moves forward, the
left hand moves down in an arc to hip level, while the right hand "stabs" forward with outstretched fingers (see photo of Form 20). Eyes are looking at the ground at 3 o'clock.

Note: Do not lean too far forward. Don't pull chin in. Left leg remains slightly bent.

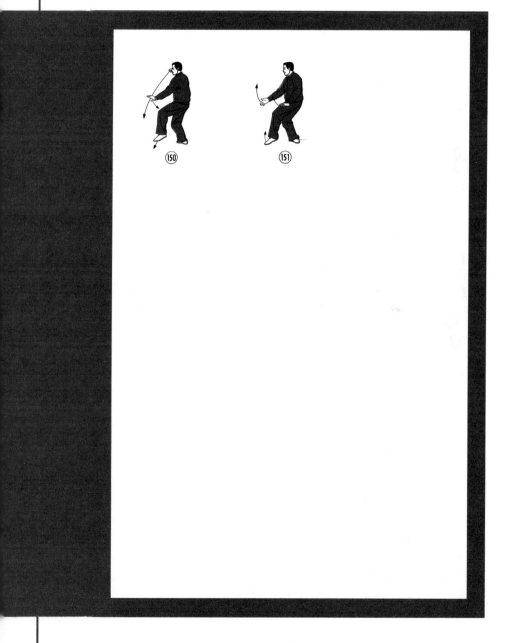

150

151

Unfolding Your Arms Like a Fan

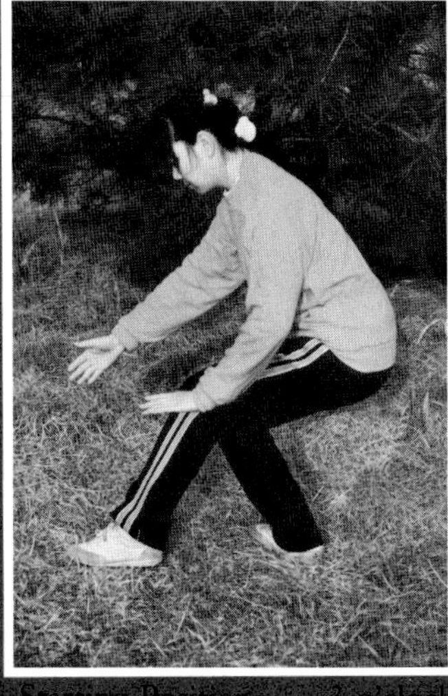

Starting Position ⟶ 3 o'clock

Weight is completely on the right leg.

152 Raise your body and turn slightly to the right to 4 o'clock; arms move up with the body.

152—154 Move right hand—by bending the elbow—up to the side of the head, turning palm of hand outward. At the same time, take a step in an arc to the left with the left leg, so that the toes point to 3 o'clock, as the left arm "stabs" forward at 3 o'clock and the weight is shifted to the left leg (left foot carries about 70 percent of the weight, the right foot about 30 percent).

Note: The arched step backwards and the arms moving in the opposite direction must be harmoniously coordinated. The left arm and left leg are on the same vertical plane exactly in the direction of the movement to 3 o'clock. The body is pointing to 4 o'clock. The distance between the two heels is about 10 to 20 cm (4 to 8 inches), which means that it is less than in the normal arched-step position.

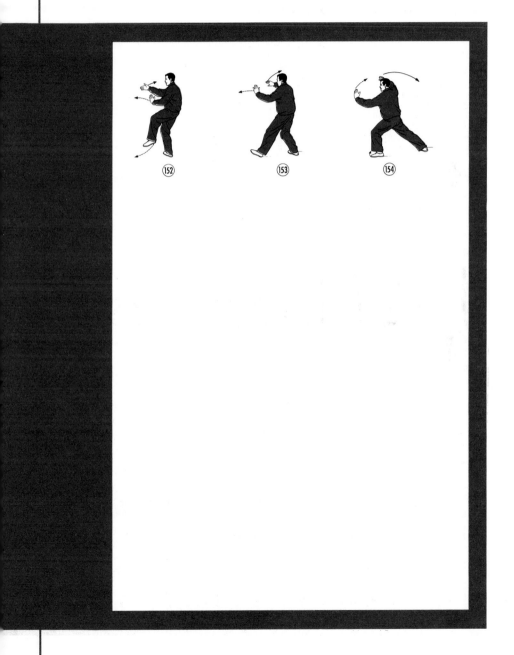
152
153
154

Turning Around, Warding Off & Punching

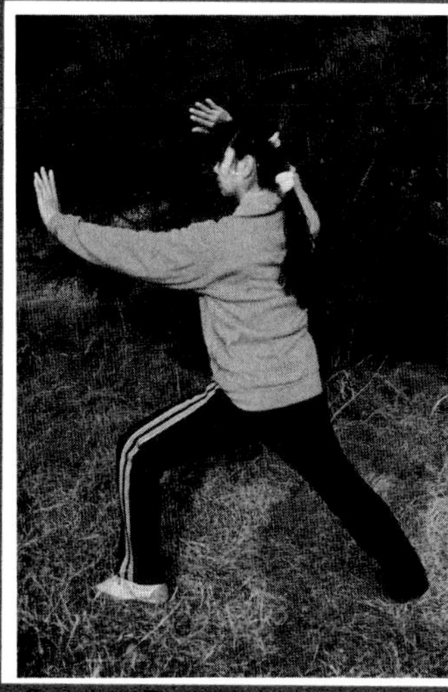

Starting Position ——→ 3 o'clock

Shift weight to the right
foot, and turn left foot
about 110 to 120° to the
inside, body and arms
155 following the rotation.
Shift weight to the left
leg, while the right hand
moves upward in an arc,
forming a fist in front of
the body at hip level
156 (fingers point to the
ground). The left arm is
rounded and follows the
upward movement to
head level; the right foot
is pulled towards the left
without touching the
ground.

Body is at 8 o'clock. Continue to turn the body to 10
o'clock, placing the right foot with a *cross-over* step at 45° to
the direction of movement, now at 9 o'clock. At the same
157 time as the body rotates and the cross step is made, the right
bent arm is straightened out and the fist is turned so that the
158 fingers point up. The left bent arm is moved down, while the
body rotates and meets the opened right hand at hip level.
The left arm is on the outside. With the full weight on the
right leg, the body continues to rotate to 11 o'clock.

The arm with the fist moves with the body rotation to the
right and back (reaching-back movement), and the left arm is
stretched out forward at 9 o'clock. With the reaching-back
movement of the right arm, the fist is turned so that the fingers are pointing to the ground; at the end of the reaching-
back movement, they point up, and when "punching"
158 forward, finally, they are on an angle facing the body. At the
time the right fist punches forward, the left leg takes an
arched step to the left, and the weight is shifted to the left
161 leg. The left arm—slightly bent—moves back, and the left
forearm touches the open right hand (161); eyes look toward
9 o'clock.

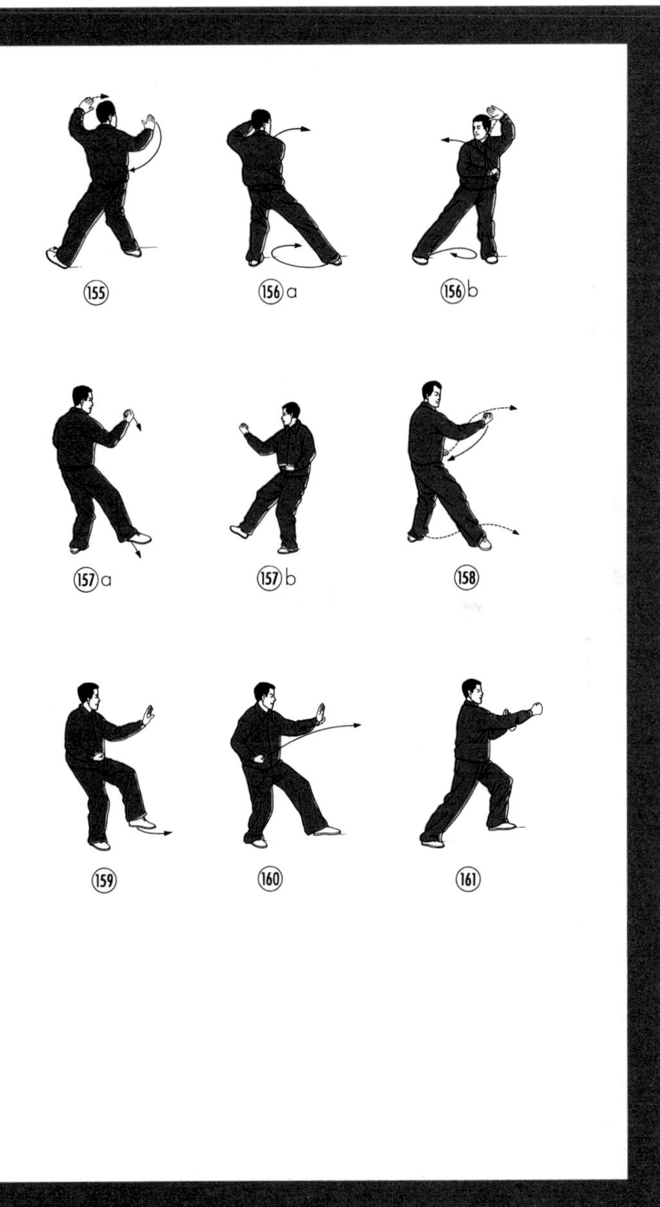
155
156a
156b
157a
157b
158
159
160
161

Closure

(162)–(163) The left hand, with the back of the hand up, crosses the right forearm behind the wrist (right hand is on top). Open fist of the right hand, and turn both hands so that both palms are pointing up.

(164)–(165) Pull hands away from each other while, at the same time, shifting the weight to the right leg and pulling the elbows towards the body. Pull hands back as if they were stroking an oval-shaped object.

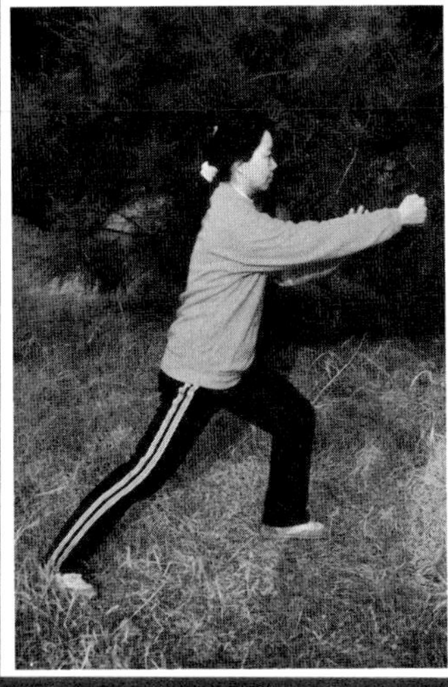

Starting Position ⟶ 9 o'clock

(166)–(167) Push forward and shift the weight to the left leg, following the sequence of movements in Form 7, (65)–(66).

Eyes are looking toward 9 o'clock.

Note: When shifting the weight to the right leg, the toes of the left foot are slightly lifted off the ground (164) and are back on the ground during the pushing movement (165)–(166).

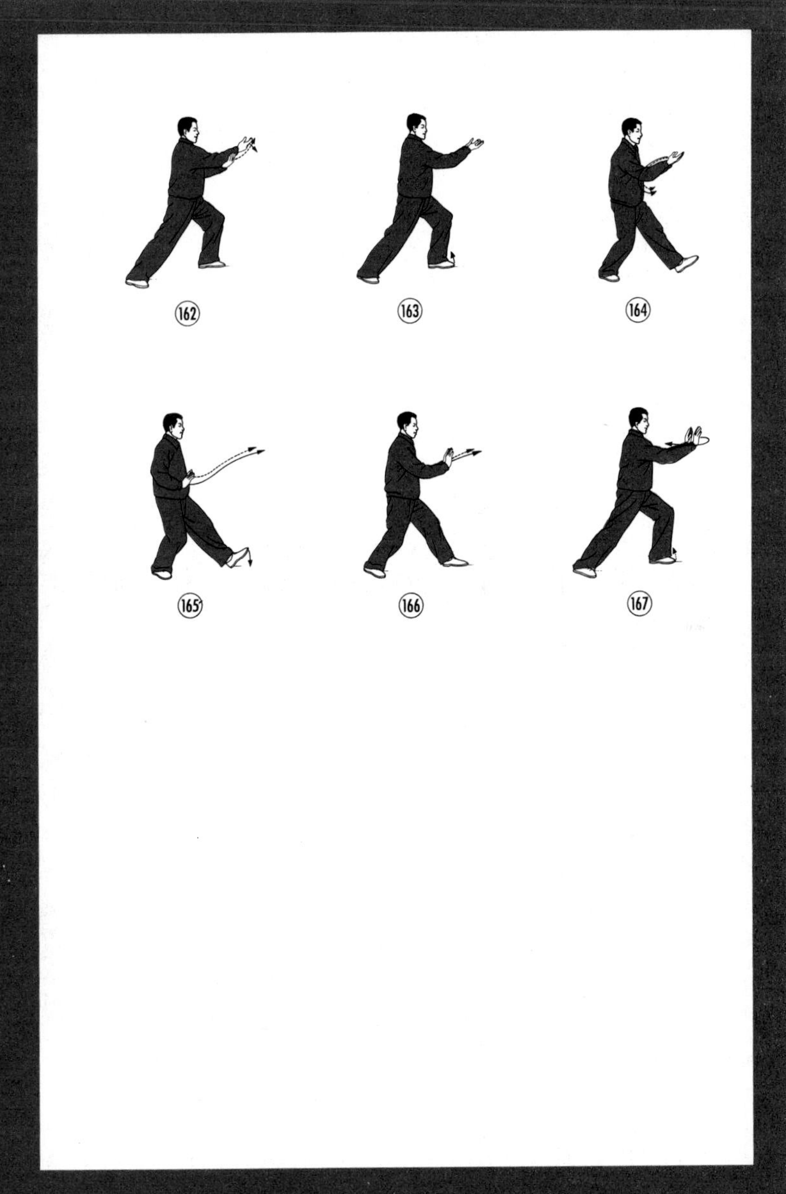

Crossing Your Hands

Shift weight back to the
right leg, and turn the
168 left foot about 90° to
the inside. After placing
170 the left foot on the
ground, immediately
rotate the right foot on
the heel so that the toes
point to about 12 to 1
o'clock.

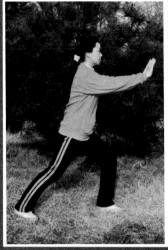

Following the rotation of the body, both hands are pulled into opposite directions at shoulder level and moved in a circle (first down and then up) until they cross each other again in front of the chest, right hand
on top. The circle per-
171 formed with the right hand is more pronounced by rotating
of the body to 1 o'clock and by briefly bending and shifting the weight to the right leg. The eyes follow the right
hand. As the right hand moves upward, the right leg is
placed—the width of a foot—parallel to the left foot.

Starting Position — 9 o'clock

Note: Do not bend the upper body forward during the circling movement of the arms; rather, lower the body slightly by bending the left knee.

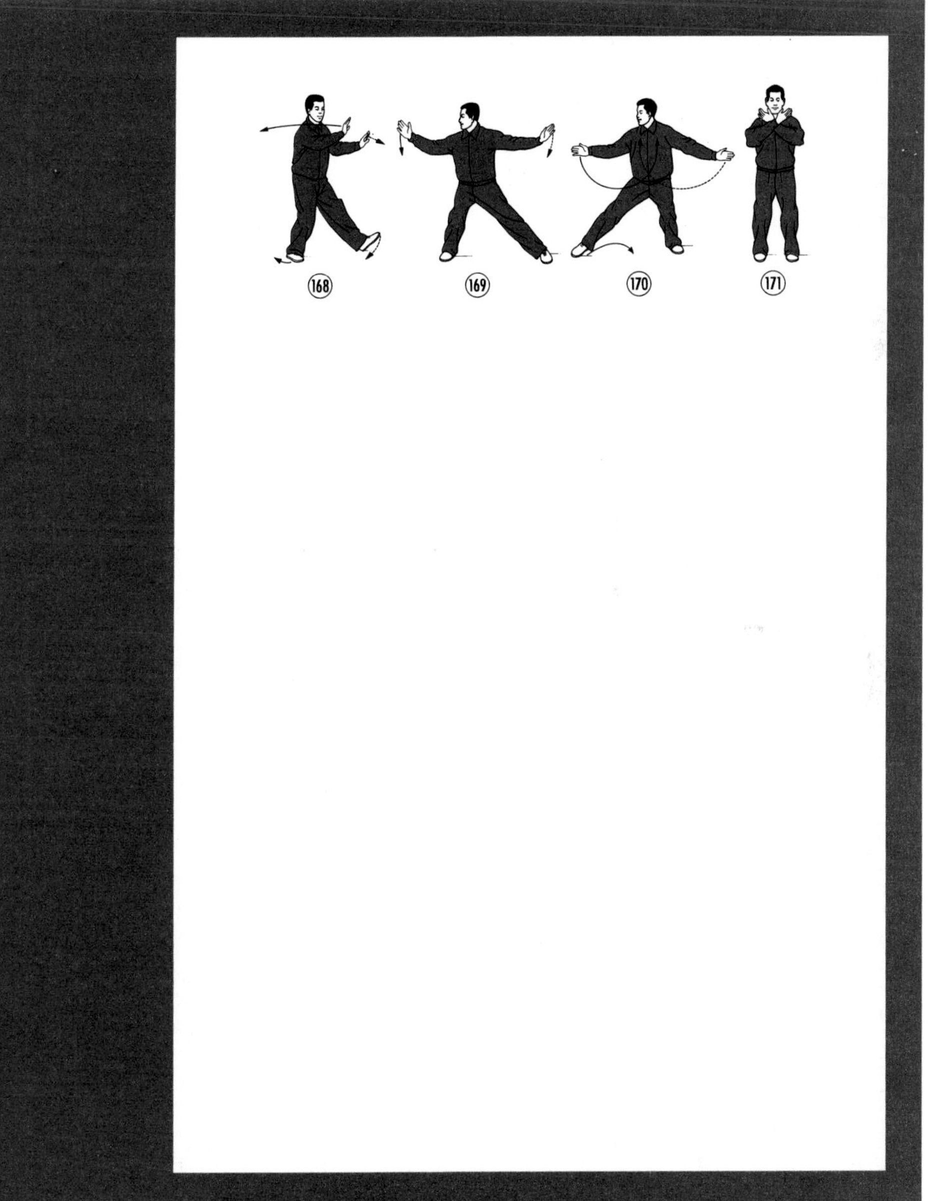

168
169
170
171

Conclusion

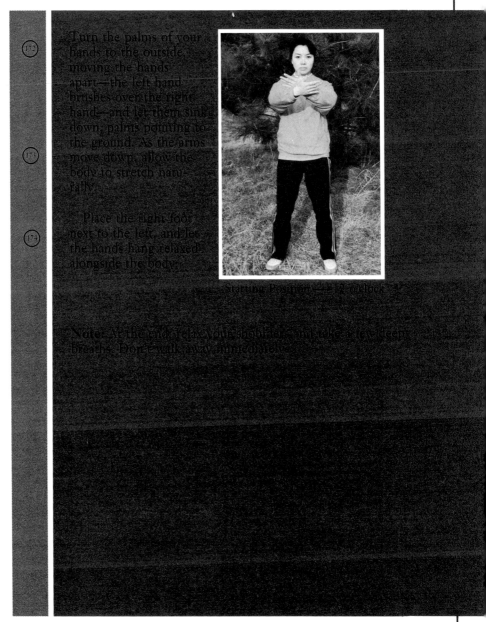

Turn the palms of your
172 hands to the outside,
moving the hands
apart—the left hand
brushes over the right
hand—and let them sink
down, palms pointing to
the ground. As the arms
173 move down, allow the
body to stretch natu-
rally.

Place the right foot
174 next to the left, and let
the hands hang relaxed
alongside the body.

Starting Position → 12 o'clock

Note: At the end, relax your shoulders and take a few deep breaths. Don't walk away immediately.

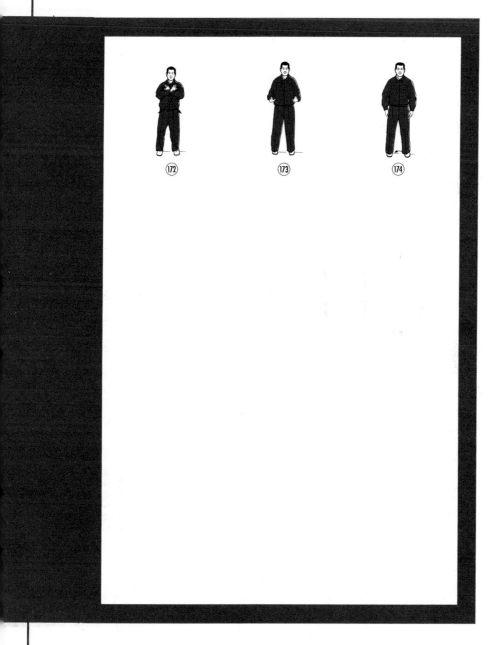

Short Glossary

These definitions refer to the terms as they are used in this book.

Beijing Short Form
This is the shortest form, put together in 1956 by the National Sports Committee of the People's Republic of China, and is based on the Yang style.

Sequence
1. The totality of certain sequences of a form.
2. Synonym for *Form* (as in Beijing Short Form).

Form
The term for a certain attack or defense movement within a Tai Chi Ch'uan sequence. Some forms consist of two or more attack and defense movements.

Short Bibliography

Capra, F. *Wendezeit.* (*Turning Point.*) Munich, 1988. Nechsel von Weich-

Chen, Y.-L. *Tai Chi Ch'uan.* Shanghai, 1943.

Engelhardt, U. *Die Klassische Tradition der Qi-Ubungen (Qigong).* (*The Classic Tradition of Qigong.*) Stuttgart, 1987.

Geissler, K. A. *Zeit leben.* (*Life to Its Fullest.*) Weinheim, Germany, 1989.

Matsui, Sugiyama, and Zhou. *On the Changing of the Heart Rate during Tai Chi Ch'uan Performance by an Expert.* Department of Physical Education, Faculty of Liberal Arts, Shizuoka University, Shizuoka, Japan, 1992.

Meinel, K., and Schnabel, G. *Bewegungslehre.* (*Theory of Movement.*) Berlin, 1987.

Pokert, M. *Die chinesische Medizin.* (*Chinese Medicine.*) Dusseldorf, 1986.

Index